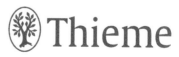

The Art of Pterygium Surgery

Mastering Techniques and Optimizing Results

Arun C. Gulani, MD, MS
Founding Director and Chief Surgeon
Gulani Vision Institute
Jacksonville, Florida

Thieme
New York • Stuttgart • Delhi • Rio de Janeiro

Library of Congress Cataloging-in-Publication Data

Names: Gulani, Arun C., editor.
Title: The art of pterygium surgery : mastering techniques and optimizing results / [edited by] Arun C. Gulani.
Description: New York : Thieme, [2020] | Includes bibliographical references. | Identifiers: LCCN 2018041472 (print) | LCCN 2018041975 (ebook) | ISBN 9781626235120 (ebook) | ISBN 9781626235113 (hardcover) | ISBN 9781626235120 (eISBN)
Subjects: | MESH: Pterygium--surgery | Ophthalmologic Surgical Procedures--methods | Postoperative Complications--prevention & control
Classification: LCC RE326.P7 (ebook) | LCC RE326.P7 (print) | NLM WW 212 | DDC 617.7/1--dc23
LC record available at https://lccn.loc.gov/2018041472

© 2020 Thieme Medical Publishers, Inc.

Thieme Publishers New York
333 Seventh Avenue, New York, NY 10001 USA
+1 800 782 3488, customerservice@thieme.com

Thieme Publishers Stuttgart
Rüdigerstrasse 14, 70469 Stuttgart, Germany
+49 [0]711 8931 421, customerservice@thieme.de

Thieme Publishers Delhi
A-12, Second Floor, Sector-2, Noida-201301
Uttar Pradesh, India
+91 120 45 566 00, customerservice@thieme.in

Thieme Publishers Rio de Janeiro, Thieme Publicações Ltda.
Edifício Rodolpho de Paoli, 25º andar
Av. Nilo Peçanha, 50 – Sala 2508,
Rio de Janeiro 20020-906 Brasil
+55 21 3172-2297 / +55 21 3172-1896
www.thiemerevinter.com.br

Cover design: Thieme Publishing Group
Typesetting by Thomson Digital, India

Printed in The United States of America
by King Printing Co., Inc.   5 4 3 2 1

ISBN 978-1-62623-511-3

Also available as an e-book:
eISBN 978-1-62623-512-0

Important note: Medicine is an ever-changing science undergoing continual development. Research and clinical experience are continually expanding our knowledge, in particular our knowledge of proper treatment and drug therapy. Insofar as this book mentions any dosage or application, readers may rest assured that the authors, editors, and publishers have made every effort to ensure that such references are in accordance with **the state of knowledge at the time of production of the book.**

Nevertheless, this does not involve, imply, or express any guarantee or responsibility on the part of the publishers in respect to any dosage instructions and forms of applications stated in the book. **Every user is requested to examine carefully** the manufacturers' leaflets accompanying each drug and to check, if necessary in consultation with a physician or specialist, whether the dosage schedules mentioned therein or the contraindications stated by the manufacturers differ from the statements made in the present book. Such examination is particularly important with drugs that are either rarely used or have been newly released on the market. Every dosage schedule or every form of application used is entirely at the user's own risk and responsibility. The authors and publishers request every user to report to the publishers any discrepancies or inaccuracies noticed. If errors in this work are found after publication, errata will be posted at www.thieme.com on the product description page.

Some of the product names, patents, and registered designs referred to in this book are in fact registered trademarks or proprietary names even though specific reference to this fact is not always made in the text. Therefore, the appearance of a name without designation as proprietary is not to be construed as a representation by the publisher that it is in the public domain.

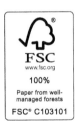

FSC
www.fsc.org
100%
Paper from well-managed forests
FSC® C103101

Contents

Contents

Video Contents

Foreword

Pterygium is a common presenting problem in every ophthalmologists practice worldwide. The pathology of a pterygium demonstrates elastotic degeneration and fibrovascular proliferation. Pterygium is more common in equatorial environments where exposure to sunshine is more intense. Blowing sand and dust can also exacerbate the incidence and prevalence of pterygium in a population. In some parts of the world I have visited, nearly every senior patient presenting for cataract surgery demonstrated pinguecula and usually at least a mild pterygium. Pterygium in emerging countries can result in significant visual loss, initially secondary to induced with the rule astigmatism, and if neglected the pterygium can invade the visual axis. In Minnesota, USA, where I live, pterygium is less prevalent but still quite common in my practice as a consultative corneal surgeon. In advanced countries, many patients seek treatment to reduce the often associated symptoms of foreign body sensation, reflex tearing, itching, and inflammation. Intermittent episodes of redness often prompt patients to seek treatment for cosmetic reasons. The eyes are critical in every cultures definition of beauty, and poor cosmesis is an important indication for pterygium surgery. Patients with pterygium will often describe being self-conscious, which can lead to social isolation and loss of confidence. Many suffer from low self-esteem and some even lapse into clinical depression. There are a diverse number of surgical approaches recommended for the removal of pterygium—all involve excision of the pterygium. The art of pterygium surgery begins *after* excision. Judgment must be exercised as to how much conjunctivae to remove, how extensive a dissection of the pathologic tenons to complete, whether or not to apply an antimetabolites such as Mitomycin C, and especially how the defect left by the surgical excision is managed. We and our patients are all striving for an excellent functional and cosmetic outcome with a minimum recurrence rate. Sometimes neglected patients desire to have a white comfortable eye as soon as possible after surgery. A superb anatomic result is of course critical, but many patients will judge the surgical outcome and the surgeon, based on the cosmetic result from day 1 postoperative. In addition, pterygium surgery is often performed prior to refractive corneal and refractive cataract surgeries. Attention to detail can enhance not only the cosmetic outcome but also offer many patients the opportunity to reduce a lifetime of dependence on spectacles. Arun C. Gulani, MD, MS, founding director and chief surgeon of the Gulani Vision Institute, has dedicated nearly three decades to perfecting an approach to pterygium surgery that generates both an excellent functional but especially a superb cosmetic outcome from day 1 postoperative. In this book, The Art of Pterygium Surgery, published by Thieme, he shares his surgical technique pearls and mindset in detail with the reader. His drive to raise pterygium and pinguecula surgery and by that effect ocular surface surgery itself to cosmetic outcomes—as well as to document postoperative patient reactions in the mirror next day after surgery along with full face photography—raises the bar on this surgical specialty not only in performance but also in expectations. In addition, this level of outcome allows many such patients who were told they are *not a candidate* for laser refractive or premium cataract surgery to become *candidates* and achieve their goals of *look good and see good.*

Toward this dedicated endeavor, Dr. Gulani has recruited a truly remarkable collection of experts from around the world to share their approaches to the management of pterygium. The techniques are discussed in detail and include the use of conjunctival autografts, amniotic membrane transplantation, antimetabolites, sutures versus fibrin glue, postoperative medical therapy, the management of complications, and the performance of follow on surgical procedures for further restoration and enhancement of vision. This is a book worthy of a place in every ophthalmologist's library.

Richard L. Lindstrom, MD
Founder and Attending Surgeon
Minnesota Eye Consultants
Adjunct Professor Emeritus
Department of Ophthalmology
University of Minnesota
Minneapolis, Minnesota
Visiting Professor
Gavin Herbert Eye Institute
University of California – Irvine
Irvine, California

Preface

Pterygium, an ocular pathology documented even in Egyptian hieroglyphics, stems from a Latinized version of the Greek term "pterygion" meaning "small wing." Mention to its management is evident in writers dating back to Sushruta, Hippocrates, Aetius, Celsus, and Pallus. In 25 AD, Celsus described his surgical approach while Sushruta as well as other learned surgeons of their times realized its misleading simplicity yet surety in frustrating recurrences.

Thousands of years later, we have still not relinquished this common, apparently simple and yet embarrassingly recurring ocular surface pathology with a high "nuisance" factor.

Further, over the years with increasing cosmetic awareness and glasses-free vision expectations, even more patients are seeking help.

This book is an attempt to take this blemish of thousands of years ago and move it into the future not only in surgical expertise and technological advances but also in patient expectations.

A stellar team of worldwide authors have put together jointly, their experience, pearls, and foresight to help the readers from all levels of eye care providers to symbiotically advance in providing a guidebook of different unbiased approaches, personal tips, and collective expectations.

Techniques of primary pterygium surgery including adjunctive use of Mitomycin C and various graft materials from conjunctival autograft to many varieties and formats of amniotic tissue with adhesive glues are all discussed in addition to correction of surgical complications and complex case managements, which include lamellar corneal surgery and even stem cell transplants to futuristic combinations of pharmaceutical, laser, and stem cell therapies.

High-impact photos, surgical videos, and tables along with online versions further underscore the impact of this new textbook on the worldwide teaching platform.

New grading systems and observation criteria and nonsurgical treatments, including specialty contact lenses, are discussed by experts to review its use before and after surgery to further enhance surgical outcomes or to compensate for induced complications or associated pathology.

I personally believe this book consolidates the past, evaluates the present, and positions for the future what I believe could be a new era for this exciting subspecialty of ocular surface surgery itself.

My Personal Journey

As I remember vividly, my first pterygium surgery was 28 years ago as a junior resident; to me it was obvious that the eye had to look perfect the next day postoperative and forever. I laboriously operated on what was considered a case for a first year resident, and I was questioned about why I took so long and what my objective was!

When I explained I was aiming for a sparkling white eye while taking all anatomic and safety precautions, I was told that it was not necessary and that prevalent dictum fuelled me to change the perspective of surgeons first and then patients, to follow.

This was similar to when I pursued refractive surgery, nearly three decades ago, where I never understood why surgeons stopped at 20/20 when my own unaided vision was 20/10; it became my dedicated focus to ensure that vision goal for every patient since.

Just as refractive surgery, where surgeons pushing for beyond 20/20 finally became a norm, I still struggled with visiting surgeons and fellows to emphasize on changing their attitude in ocular surface surgery to deliver symptom-free aesthetics and safe long-term impact, with finally tying this outcome to assure refractive surgery candidacy as a birthright for every human being to have a perfect vision as well as to look good, without compromising either.

As I have always said to surgeons I train, "Your hands cannot do what your mind has not decided," and hence I enforce an attitude first, followed by surgical skills that automatically result in outcomes, which surgeons and their patients can celebrate enthusiastically.

In fact, in my initial days, I was so surprised with the consistency of my day 1 postoperative outcomes— ecstatic patient responses in addition to the respectful disbelief of visiting surgeons, industry representatives, and thousands of attendees in worldwide audiences where I lectured— that I took it on myself to make my work so accountable, as if I was looking for a fault, that I could report to finally satisfy my able colleagues and the industry itself.

Hence, I went overboard in recoding surgeries, day 1 postoperative, and further follow-up visit photos— photos beyond just eyes, showing patient's faces and their true delight as well as video recordings of in the mirror patient responses when seeing their own operated eyes day 1 postsurgery for the first time. I would personally follow-up on patients (maximum follow-up being 16 years) and insist on asking about pain, discomfort, feelings about their eye appearance, and they would in excitement and thankfulness want pictures with me that they could proudly share with family and friends worldwide.

I made it my accountability adage, "I cannot think of a higher accountability than having my surgical patient on camera stating their experience without a script, makeup, or incentive."

When my success drew patients not only with pterygium but also with pinguecula (cosmetic level) from around the world, I would sit and reason with them initially until I compiled a list of symptoms they commonly shared—besides them flying to me from different countries, cultures, and geographic locales.

I listed these in escalating order right from such patients being "self-conscious, to having low self-esteem, to being depressed as the final end of that spectrum." I initially saw movie stars, models, and news anchors and then women, more than men, with pinguecula started seeking my services and then over the years I see everyday people from all walks of life came to see me and the number of males seeking this correction has been rising.

To keep my excitement separate from my integrity —though I was a believer in what I was doing and selflessly sharing with colleagues worldwide—I never made any deals or advertised or lured any patient. I would operate only after they signed extensive informed consents that made it clear that this was a serious surgery and there were no guarantees for outcomes. I in fact listed all kinds of complications that could occur and only after such a strict informed consent, would I agree to operate on patients.

With such levels of integrity—despite my successful results that drew patients from all over the world— I also made it personal to follow-up till date with my patients (who developed less than desired outcomes) and/or with their respective eye doctors to the best of my ability.

In this book, therefore, I have included my endeavors of over 28 years toward innovating, documenting, and teaching along with a stellar co-faculty of authors whose surgical skills and reputations stand out as among the best in the world so we could also provide a diverse viewpoint and experience to the readers in an effort to allow them to contribute, perform, adapt, and even challenge us toward our common goal in raising pterygium surgery to an art.

Arun C. Gulani

Acknowledgments

I would first like to thank my patients from all over the world who allow me to execute my passion in reciprocation for their trust. It's their blessings and encouragement that continue to fuel my endeavor.

I would like to thank my family: my parents, my siblings, my children, Aaisha and Yash, and my beloved wife, Suparna, for their unfailing support and understanding my commitment of time and effort to make this book into a reality.

Thanks to my staff for their patience as we documented all levels of preoperative and postoperative data, personalized care for each patient, and then recorded all patients, live videos, photos, and patient reactions for all our patients, as part of our practice mission.

I would like to acknowledge and thank my coauthors—stellar surgeons and renowned global authorities who shared their diverse experiences to enrich this book. They took pride in contributing to this book in believing and then creating it to be the next generation of teaching in this subspecialty.

Thank you Dr. Eric Donnefeld, Dr. Scheffer Tseng, Dr. Hank Perry, Dr. Amar Agarwal, Dr. Soosan Jacob, Dr. Virendra Sanwan, Dr. Ashvin Agarwal, Dr. Boris Malyugin, Dr. Alan Carlson, Dr. Jorge Alio, Dr. Minas Corneo, Dr. Eduardo Alphanso, Dr. Ming Wang, Dr. Sonal Tuli, Dr. Paul Karpecki, Dr. Nathan Schramm, Dr. Andy Morgenstern, Dr. Tom Arnold, and Dr. Christine Sindt.

I would like to thank thousands of eye surgeons (visiting surgeons, fellows, residents, attendees) over the last three decades who in the garb of learning from me actually inspired and catapulted my desire to excel and hold myself accountable to them all.

My respectful thanks to my esteemed colleagues, who travelled to witness my work and provided legitimate reason for me to believe that this work is indeed the future.

My heartfelt thanks to Bill Lamsback and the entire team at Theime publishers for realizing my endeavor in print to bring out a spectacular product in tune with present times and technology to best reach all levels of eye care providers in the name of education.

I would also like to thank, in anticipation, the readers, ranging across all levels of eye care providers. Hopefully you can carry the baton forward and even add or improve this text for the next edition.

Last but not the least, thanks to Dick Lindstrom who consolidated his verbal expression for my work and established its position in the world of eye surgery.

Contributors

Ahmed A. Abdelghany, MD
Lecturer
Ophthalmology Department
Faculty of Medicine
Minia University Hospital
Minia, Egypt

Amar Agarwal, MS, FRCS, FRCOphth
Professor
Chairman
Dr. Agarwal's Group of Eye Hospitals
Past President
ISRS/AAO
Secretary General
Indian Intraocular Implant and Refractive Surgery
Chennai, Tamil Nadu, India

Ashvin Agarwal, MS
Executive Director
Dr Agarwal's Eye Hospital and Eye Research Center
Chennai, Tamil Nadu, India

Eduardo Alfonso, MD
Director, Bascom Palmer Eye Institute
Chairman, Department of Ophthalmology
Kathleen and Stanley Glaser Professor
University of Miami
Miami, Florida

Jorge L. Alio, MD, PhD
Professor and Chairman of Ophthalmology
Miguel Hernández University
Edificio Vissum, Alicante, Spain

Nancy Argano, OD
Optometrist
Eye Physicians of Central Jersey
Old Bridge, New Jersey

Thomas P. Arnold, OD, FSLS
President
Today's Vision Sugar Land
Sugar Land, Texas

Melissa Barnett, OD, FAAO, FSLS, FBCLA
Principal Optometrist
University of California Davis Eye Center
Sacramento, California

Alan N. Carlson, MD
Professor
Department of Ophthalmology
Duke University School of Medicine
Durham, North Carolina

Anny M.S. Cheng, MD
Clinical Assistant Professor
Ocular Surface Center
Miami, Florida
Florida International University
Herbert Wertheim College of Medicine
Miami, Florida

Ilan Cohen, MD
Cornea Specialist
Eye Physicians of Central Jersey
Old Bridge, New Jersey

Minas T. Coroneo, MD, MD, MSc
Professor and Chairman
Department of Ophthalmology, University of New South Wales, Sydney at Prince of Wales Hospital, Randwick
Ophthalmic Surgeons, Sydney
Look for Life Foundation
East Sydney Private Hospital, Sydney
Randwick, NSW, Australia

Eric D. Donnenfeld, MD, FACS
Cornea, Laser, Cataract, and Refractive Surgeon
OCLI
Garden City, New York

Aaishwariya A. Gulani, BS
Wharton School of Business
University of Pennsylvania
Philadelphia, Pennsylvania

Arun C. Gulani, MD
Founding Director and Chief Surgeon
Gulani Vision Institute
Jacksonville, Florida

Soosan Jacob, MS, FRCS, DNB
Director and Chief
Dr. Agarwal's Eye Hospital and Eye Research Center
Chennai, Tamil Nadu, India

Dhivya Ashok Kumar, MD, FRCS, FICO, FAICO
Senior Consultant and Head R&D
Dr. Agarwal's Eye Hospital and Eye Research Centre
Chennai, Tamil Nadu, India

Abhinav Loomba, MS
Clinical Research Ophthalmologist
Department of Cornea and Anterior Segment Services
Department of Tele-ophthalmology
LV Prasad Eye Institute
Banjara Hills, Hyderabad, India

Andrew S. Morgenstern, OD, FAAO
Assistant Professor
Uniformed Services University
Department of Surgery
Walter Reed National Military Medical Center
Bethesda, Maryland

Alanna S. Nattis DO
Cornea, Cataract, and Refractive Surgeon
Director of Clinical Research
Lindenhurst Eye Physicians and Surgeons
Babylon, New York
Associate Professor of Ophthalmology and Surgery
College of Osteopathic Medicine
New York Institute of Technology
Glen Head, New York

Sotiria Palioura, MD
Voluntary Assistant Professor of Ophthalmology
Bascom Palmer Eye Institute
University of Miami Miller School of Medicine
Miami, Florida

Parth G. Patel, MD
Consultant - Cornea and Anterior Segment Surgeon
PBMA's Kantai Netralaya
Mumbai, Maharashtra, India

Henry D. Perry, MD
Professor of Ophthalmology
Hofstra University
Nassau University Medical Center
Ophthalmic Consultants of Long Island
East Meadow, New York

Nathan Rock, OD, FAAO
Consultative Optometrist
Wang Vision Cataract & LASIK Center – An Aier-USA
    Eye Clnic
Nashville, Tennessee

Virender Singh Sangwan, MS
Director
Center for Ocular Regeneration
Dr Paul Dubord Chair in Cornea
Tej Kohli Cornea Institute
LV Prasad Eye Institute
Hyderabad, India

Nathan Schramm, OD, FSLS, CNS
Optometric Physician
Natural Eyes of Weston
Fort Lauderdale, Florida

Christine W. Sindt, OD, FAAO
Director
Contact Lens Service
Clinical Professor of Ophthalmology and Visual
    Sciences
Iowa City, Iowa

Tracy Schroeder Swartz, OD, MS, FAAO, DIPL ABO
Optometrist
Madison Eye Care Center
Madison, Alabama

Scheffer C.G. Tseng, MD, PhD
Medical Director
Ocular Surface Center
Miami, Florida

Sonal Tuli, MD, MEd
Professor and Chair
Department of Ophthalmology
University of Florida
Gainesville, Florida

Ming Wang, MD, PhD
CEO
Aier-USA
Clinical Professor
Meharry Medical College
Director
Wang Vision Cataract & LASIK Center
Nashville, Tennessee

1 Pterygium: History and Overview

Arun C. Gulani and Parth G. Patel

Abstract

One of the oldest pathologies in eye care has today reached a cosmetic level of surgical outcomes due to better understanding of the pathophysiology and technological advances in surgical applications to address raised patient expectations.

Keywords: pterygium surgery, SPARKLE pterygium technique, no-stitch pterygium surgery, fibrin glue, amniotic graft

1.1 Introduction

Pterygium is a common disease of the eye and has been described in medical and surgical texts since as long back as 1000 BC.[1] The word "pterygium" stems from the Greek word "pterygos," which means "wing" (plural: pterygia), and is an accurate description of its appearance. The pterygium has been defined as a triangular, wing-shaped, degenerative, fibrovascular, hyperplastic proliferative tissue actively growing from the conjunctival limbal area onto the cornea.[2] It is an external, superficial, elevated ocular mass that forms over the perilimbal conjunctiva and extends onto the corneal surface. It continues to grow to cover the center of the cornea, usually from the nasal side, but may come from the temporal side or rarely from both.

1.2 Epidemiology

The incidence of pterygium has been directly linked to proximity to the equator. The latitudes between 37 degree north and south of the equator were referred to as the "pterygium belt" by Cameron.[3] Increasing age, ultraviolet (UV) radiation, chronic irritation, and genetic predisposition are the other risk factors.

1.3 Pathophysiology

The exact cause or mechanism of pterygium formation is still unknown. They are thought to be a degenerative process caused by sun exposure and show altered collagen fibers with elastic stains, classically described as "elastotic degeneration."[4] Newer studies hint toward pterygium being a localized, interpalpebral, limbal stem cell deficiency due to exposure to UV radiation.[5]

1.4 History

The first description of pterygium and the surgical procedure to treat it was given by Sushruta, probably the world's first surgeon ophthalmologist, who lived in India around 1000 BC. Since then, there have been many descriptions by Celsus (29 AD), Vagblat and Paul (600 AD), Rhazes (932 AD), Avicenna (1037 AD), and Chakradatta (1060 AD).[6]

Since the beginning, the preferred mode of treatment was surgical, although many medical treatments have also been tried.

The ancient Egyptians used "collyria" of pastes of honey, excrement of lizard or pelican, incense, or antimony to treat many eye diseases including pterygia.[7] Hippocrates (V–IV centuries BC) mentioned collyria of zinc, copper, iron, bile, urine, and mother's milk.[8] Centuries later, Bartisch[9] and Sennert[10] recommended a mixture of sugar, bloodstone (hematite powder), alum, white vitriol, camphor, and wine tartar. A classical treatment was Divine Stone (lapis divinus, also called lapis ophthalmicus), which was a mixture of potassium nitrate, alum, blue vitriol, and camphor dissolved in water.[11]

The oldest preserved surgical description, that of Sushruta, describes the surgery as follows (▶ Fig. 1.1):

"The patient must lie on a table. The pterygium is sprinkled with salt. The patient looks laterally, and the most superficial part of the pterygium is clasped with a hook. Then, the pterygium is detached from the ocular surface with a knife with a round end but sharp cutting edge. The remnants adhered to the eye must be eliminated, and an unguent applied, in order to avoid the recurrence."[12]

Celsus used a thread under the pterygium instead of a hook and cut the detached pterygium with a scalpel. He then placed a cloth soaked in honey on the surface.[13] The centuries that followed saw many of the surgeons using their own modifications of this technique.

Modern approach to treatment includes using ocular lubricants to treat dry eye during the early stages of the disease. Surgical treatment is conventionally indicated when the lesion is large, threatens vision, causes significant discomfort, or is cosmetically unacceptable. Surgical methods include a wide range of procedures from the simple bare sclera

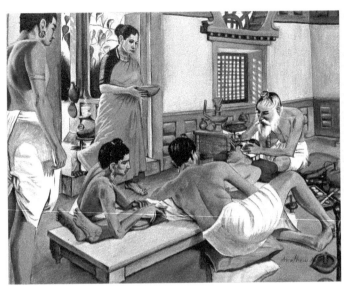

Fig. 1.1 Depiction of Sushruta during his surgeries. (Reproduced with permission from Dr. Babu Thushar.)

technique to the more complex lamellar kerato-plasty and amniotic membrane transplantation. All these techniques aim to minimize recurrence, which is the biggest problem encountered in treating pterygia.

The current surgical approaches can broadly be divided into the following[14]:
1. Bare sclera excision.
2. Excision with conjunctival closure.
3. Excision with antimitotic adjunctive therapies.
4. Ocular surface transplantation techniques.

The bare sclera technique, which was first described by D'Ombrain in 1948,[15] is now out of favor due to the high incidence of recurrence.[16] Excision with a simple conjunctival closure is popularly performed in developing countries. It includes a range of techniques like simple approximation of the conjunctival edges to superior rotational flap transposition. This reduces the recurrence.[17] There is widespread acceptance of conjunctival autografting, since it was introduced by Thoft (1977) and was applied to pterygium surgery by Vastine et al and Kenyon et al.[18] Most techniques advocate using an adequately sized thin graft devoid of Tenon's fascia to cover the bare sclera. Closure can be achieved by either sutures or adhesives. Fibrin glue is the most common adhesive currently used. It is biodegradable and induces very little inflammatory reaction.

Many adjunctive therapies have been used to reduce the rate of recurrence, none without their own complications. These include the following:
1. Corticosteroids: After pterygium excision, topical corticosteroids diminish the tissue reaction and inflammation and, consequently, the danger of recurrences. They are now accepted as the normal protocol after pterygium surgery.[19]
2. Thiotepa (triethylene thiophosphoramide): It is a radiomimetic agent that obliterates neovessels by inhibiting mitosis of the endothelium of the capillaries. Diluted thiotepa (1:2,000) is used topically. Complications include vasodilatation of the conjunctival vessels, allergy to thiotepa, and depigmentation of the lid skin.[20]
3. Cyclosporin A: It inhibits calcineurin, which is a serine/threonine phosphatase that dephosphorylates the nuclear factors of activated T cells. It has an antiproliferative action on the fibroblasts of the pterygium.[21]
4. Mitomycin C (MMC): It is an antibiotic and antitumoral agent that inhibits ribonucleic acid (RNA) and deoxyribonucleic acid (DNA), the synthesis of proteins, and cellular proliferation. At 0.02% dilution, MMC has been applied with a soaked sponge to the denuded corneosclera for 2 minutes. MMC has also been used twice a day postoperatively for 5 days. Possible complications of MMC include epithelial keratopathy punctata, limbal avascularity,

scleral and corneal dystrophy, corneal decompensation, calcification plaques, and, rarely, keratomalacia (corneal melting), glaucoma, and cataract.[22] It is currently commonly used by surgeons worldwide.

5. 5-Fluorouracil (5-FU): It is a chemotherapeutic agent that inhibits thymidylate synthetase, an important enzyme for the synthesis of DNA. When a pterygium is recurring, the injection of 5-FU reduces its neovascularization, maybe because it inhibits the fibroblasts and, therefore, the consumption of oxygen and the stimulation of neovessels.[23]

6. Vascular endothelial growth factor (VEGF) inhibitors: Pterygia show high levels of proangiogenic factors, such as tumor necrosis factor (TNF)-α, VEGF, fibroblast growth factor (FGF)-2, heparin-binding epidermal growth factor (HB-EGF), interleukin (IL)-6, IL-8, and matrix metalloproteinases (MMPs). This causes the typical neovascularization of pterygium. This forms the basis of use of anti-VEGF agents, such as bevacizumab.[24]

7. Interferons (IFNs): They are cytokines secreted by cells stressed by infection, cancer, and other conditions. IFN type I (IFN-α and IFN-β) are secreted in all somatic cells, and IFN type II (IFN-γ) are secreted in the cells of the immune system. IFN-α_{2b} has been used in recurrent pterygia.[25]

8. Beta irradiation: It inhibits division of rapidly dividing cells and has thus been tried to reduce recurrence. The complications include scleral necrosis and melting, iris atrophy and cataract formation.

Last, amniotic membrane transplantation after pterygium excision is a common procedure nowadays, especially in cases of recurrent pterygia. Amniotic membrane has little antigenicity and, therefore, does not provoke immune rejection. It has leukotrienes, prostaglandins, interleukins, enzymes, epithelial growth factors, and vitamins that help normalize the ocular surface. It also has anti-VEGF, which inhibits neovascularization. It prevents fibroblastic proliferation and excessive scarring.[26] The latest advances in techniques which involve No stitches and No cutting[27] have made it possible to carry out the surgery (Gulani SPARKLE technique: Sutureless Pterygium with Amniotic Reconstruction and Lamellar Keratectomy Excision) inducing only minimal change in refraction. This is especially important in today's times, where many patients wanting to undergo pterygium surgery have had refractive surgeries in the past (▶ Fig. 1.2, ▶ Fig. 1.3, ▶ Fig. 1.4).

Today with the latest advances in medical and surgical resources, the main aim of pterygium surgery is not only to prevent recurrence but also to make the eye as aesthetically pleasing as possible. These cosmetic outcomes can be achieved by delicate and precise surgical techniques which reduce the inflammation and hasten healing. The recurrence rates have been tremendously reduced with certain studies reporting even lesser than 0.5% recurrence rate with a 16-year follow-up and that too with cosmetically pleasing results (▶ Fig. 1.5 and ▶ Fig. 1.6).[28] Advances in molecular biology have identified factors such as HC-HA/PTX3 in amniotic membrane being responsible for its anti-inflammatory effects. These advances could pave the way to using such targeted molecular-based therapeutics in the future to promote the regenerative healing in pterygium surgery.[29]

Despite this rich plethora of medical and surgical techniques, pterygium remains a common eye disease worldwide. Let us conclude with what Rosenthal has aptly said, "Down through history there were many who practiced and reported upon various operative techniques without making any outstanding contributions. They number in hundreds and their names may be found in the literature of all nations and all ages. And so it appears that for 30 centuries man has tried to conquer this little growth called pterygium. It has been incised, removed, split, galvanized, heated, dissected, rotated, coagulated, repositioned and irradiated. It has been analyzed statistically, geographically, etiologically, microscopically and chemically—yet it grows onward primarily and secondarily. We look with interest to its future."[30]

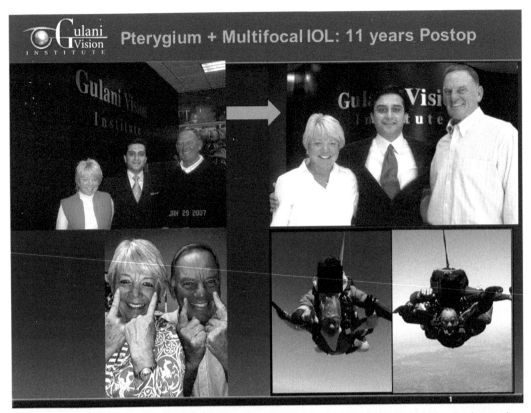

Fig. 1.2 This active couple underwent SPARKLE Pterygium surgery to a cosmetic outcome which also simultaneously restored their corneal irregularity to a smooth measurable refraction to confidently then undergo Premium Cataract surgery with Multifocal Lens implants to 20/20 vision and actively pursuing life's many sporty endeavors.

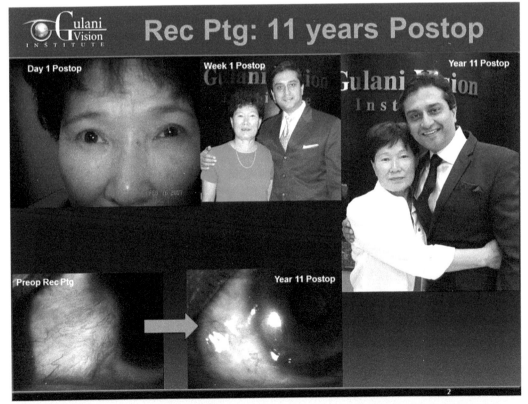

Fig. 1.3 A patient who was referred with an aggressive, recurrent pterygium and underwent SPARKLE technique to an immediate and long term cosmetic outcome and continues to enjoy her appearance over a decade later.

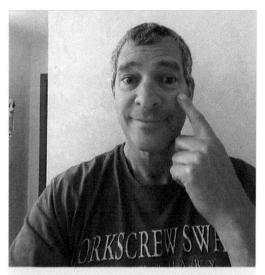

Fig. 1.4 An active young man who is a professional sportsman and musician enjoying his cosmetic outcome from day 1 to 14 years postop.

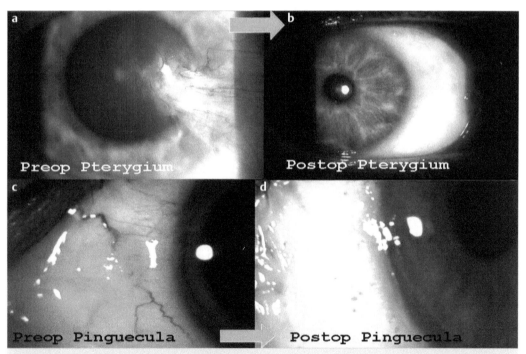

Fig. 1.5 (a-d) "Next Day" cosmetic outcomes of Gulani SPARKLE technique. SPARKLE, Sutureless Pterygium with Amniotic Reconstruction and Lamellar Keratectomy Excision.

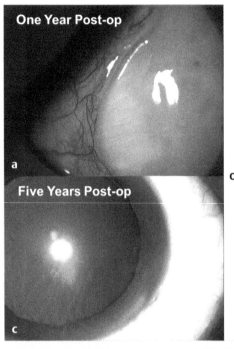
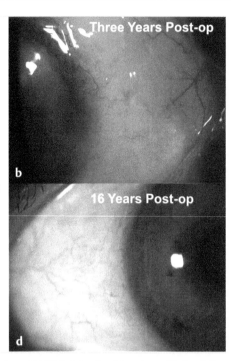

Fig. 1.6 (a-d) Long-term clinical outcomes of Gulani SPARKLE technique. SPARKLE, Sutureless Pterygium with Amniotic Reconstruction and Lamellar Keratectomy Excision.

References

[1] Coster D. Pterygium–an ophthalmic enigma. Br J Ophthalmol. 1995; 79(4):304–305

[2] Yanoff M, Duker JS. Ophthalmology. 2nd ed. Philadelphia, PA: Elsevier Publications; 2008

[3] Cameron ME. Pterygium Throughout the World. Springfield, IL: Charles C. Thomas; 1965

[4] Chui JJY, Coroneo MT. Pterygium pathogenesis, actinic damage, and recurrence. In: Hovanesian JA, ed. Pterygium: Techniques and Technologies for Surgical Success. Thorofare, NJ: Slack Incorporated; 2012:1–26

[5] Coroneo MT, Di Girolamo N, Wakefield D. The pathogenesis of pterygia. Curr Opin Ophthalmol. 1999; 10(4):282–288

[6] Johnson RD, Pai VC, Hoft RH. Historical approaches to pterygium surgery, including bare sclera and adjunctive beta radiation techniques. In: Hovanesian JA, ed. Pterygium: Techniques and Technologies for Surgical Success. Vol. 2012. Thorofare, NJ: Slack Incorporated; 2012:27–36

[7] Albert DM, Edwards DD. The History of Ophthalmology. Cambridge MA: Black-well; 1996

[8] Rojas Álvarez E.. Surgery of pterygium. A history that does not end [in Spanish]. Arch Soc Espan Oftalmol. 2008; 83: 333–33–4

[9] Bartisch von Königsbrück G. Ophthalm-odouleia, das ist Augendienst. Dresden: Mathes Stöckel; 1583

[10] Sennet D. Medicinae practicae libri VI. 1st ed. Wittenberg; 1628 1

[11] Saint-Yves C. Nouveau traité des maladies des yeux. Amsterdam & Leipzik, Arkstée & Merkus; 1767

[12] Bidyadhar NK. Susruta and his ophthalmic operations. Arch Ophthalmol. 1939; 22:550

[13] Celsus. Aulus Cornelius. De re medica [On medicine]. Circa 30–35 AD. Liber VII, 7. Published in Vol III of the Loeb Classical Library. Harvard. University Press; 1935

[14] Singh G. Pterygium and its surgery. Smolin and Thoft's The Cornea: Scientific Foundations and Clinical Practice. Philadelphia: Lippincott Williams & Wilkins; 2004.

[15] D'Ombrain A. The surgical treatment of pterygium. Br J Ophthalmol. 1948; 32(2):65–71

[16] Hirst LW. The treatment of pterygium. Surv Ophthalmol. 2003; 48(2):145–180

[17] Kamel S. Pterygium. Its nature and a new line of treatment. Br J Ophthalmol. 1946; 30:549–564

[18] Kenyon KR, Wagoner MD, Hettinger ME. Conjunctival autograft transplantation for advanced and recurrent pterygium. Ophthalmology. 1985; 92(11):1461–1470

[19] King JH , Jr. The pterygium; brief review and evaluation of certain methods of treatment. AMA Arch Opthalmol. 1950; 44(6):854–869

[20] Cassady JR. The inhibition of pterygium recurrence by thiotepa. Am J Ophthalmol. 1966; 61(5 Pt 1):886–888

[21] Turan-Vural E, Torun-Acar B, Kivanc SA, Acar S. The effect of topical 0.05% cyclosporine on recurrence following pterygium surgery. Clin Ophthalmol. 2011; 5(1):881–885

[22] Calişkan S, Orhan M, Irkeç M. Intraoperative and postoperative use of mitomycin-C in the treatment of primary pterygium. Ophthalmic Surg Lasers. 1996; 27(7):600–604

[23] Bekibele CO, Baiyeroju AM, Olusanya BA, Ashaye AO, Oluleye TS. Pterygium treatment using 5-FU as adjuvant treatment compared to conjunctiva autograft. Eye (Lond). 2008; 22(1):31–34

[24] Enkvetchakul O, Thanathanee O, Rangsin R, Lekhanont K, Suwan-Apichon O. A randomized controlled trial of intralesional bevacizumab injection on primary pterygium: preliminary results. Cornea. 2011; 30(11):1213–1218

[25] Di Girolamo N, Chui J, Coroneo MT, Wakefield D. Pathogenesis of pterygia: role of cytokines, growth factors, and matrix metalloproteinases. Prog Retin Eye Res. 2004; 23 (2):195–228

[26] Tananuvat N, Martin T. The results of amniotic membrane transplantation for primary pterygium compared with conjunctival autograft. Cornea. 2004; 23(5):458–463

[27] Gulani AC. No Stitch pterygium surgery: Next day cosmetic outcomes. Video J Ophthalmol. 2009

[28] Gulani AC, Patel PG. Raising the bar on pterygium surgery - the no stitch, no patch, no red approach. Adv Med Biol. 2017; 98:127–139

[29] He H, Zhang S, Tighe S, Son J, Tseng SC. Immobilized heavy chain-hyaluronic acid polarizes lipopolysaccharide-activated macrophages toward M2 phenotype. J Biol Chem. 2013; 288 (36):25792–25803

[30] Rosenthal JW. Chronology of pterygium therapy. Am J Ophthalmol. 1953; 36(11):1601–1616

2 Classic Signs, Symptoms, Classification, and Differential Diagnosis of Pterygium

Sotiria Palioura and Eduardo Alfonso

Abstract

Herein, we present the classic clinical signs and symptoms of pterygium lesions along with the major classification system for such lesions. We further elaborate on the differential diagnosis for pterygium, which includes pannus, pseudopterygium, and ocular surface squamous neoplasia (OSSN). Pterygium is a triangular fibrovascular tissue that extends from the bulbar conjunctiva onto the cornea within the interpalpebral fissure. Diagnosis is made by slit-lamp examination. High-resolution optical coherence tomography can aid in diagnosis of atypical pterygium lesions and is particularly useful at differentiating benign lesions from neoplastic ones. Unless inflamed, pterygia are typically asymptomatic. Progressive pterygia may affect vision either by inducing astigmatism or by obscuring the visual axis. Though there is no global consensus for the classification of pterygium lesions, intense redness, increased vascularity, and significant fleshiness represent aggressive lesions.

Keywords: pterygium, pseudopterygium, ocular surface squamous neoplasia

2.1 Introduction

Pterygium is a wing-shaped ocular surface lesion traditionally described as encroachment of fibrovascular tissue from the bulbar conjunctiva onto the cornea. Despite advances to understand the pathogenesis of pterygium, it remains a matter of debate whether it is a degenerative elastotic lesion or it represents a proliferative disorder due to an abnormal wound healing response.[1] The association of pterygia with other sun-related disorders such as cataracts, pinguecula, and ocular surface squamous neoplasia (OSSN) and their higher incidence in latitudes close to the equator suggest a major role for ultraviolet (UV) radiation in their pathogenesis.[2] Pterygia only present in humans and not in nonhuman primates or other animals, possibly due to the unique ocular morphology of humans.[3] They do have a predilection for the nasal limbus that may be explained by the phenomenon of peripheral light focusing, whereby incidental light passes through the anterior chamber and focuses at the nasal limbus, thus damaging the limbal stem cells in that area.[4]

2.2 Clinical Signs

Clinically, pterygia typically present as a triangular fleshy tissue that comes from the bulbar conjunctiva and grows onto the cornea within the interpalpebral fissure. The apex of the triangular tissue (or head of the pterygium) is found on the cornea, and the base of the triangle (or body of the pterygium) is on the bulbar conjunctiva. In the vast majority of cases, the diagnosis can be easily made upon slit-lamp examination. A characteristic straightening of the vessels in the direction of the advancing head of the pterygium on the corneal surface is also seen (▶ Fig. 2.1). A pterygium may be like a thin translucent membrane or significantly thickened with an elevated mound of gelatinous material (▶ Fig. 2.2). Depending on its vascularity, it may be white, pink, or red.

In its early stages, a pterygium is a fine transparent tissue with minimal elevation, few vessels, and very little corneal involvement. As the lesion advances, it becomes a thick opaque vascular tissue that may extend even up to the visual axis (▶ Fig. 2.3). The presence of an epithelial iron line, called Stocker's line, in front of the pterygium head suggests chronicity of the lesion. Other sun-related lesions, such as pinguecula, are present in the ipsilateral or contralateral eye. It is very unusual for pterygia to present in locations other than the 3 or 9 o'clock positions within the palpebral fissure. In fact, pterygium-looking lesions in other locations should immediately raise suspicion for alternate diagnosis.

2.3 Symptoms

Most often pterygia are asymptomatic, though many patients will admit that they are bothered by the cosmetic appearance of the lesion when asked directly. A pterygium can become inflamed and cause significant irritation and foreign body sensation. As the lesion progresses onto the surface of the cornea, it may affect vision either by obscuring the visual axis or by inducing significant

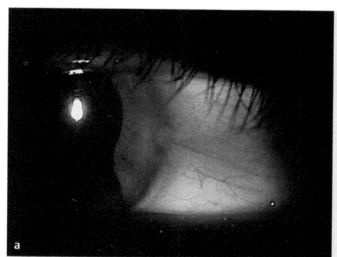

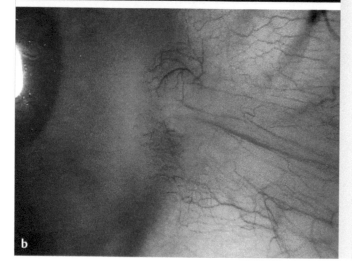

Fig. 2.1 (a) Typical pterygium with characteristic straightening of the vessels toward the advancing head. (b) Close-up view of the same lesion shows that the underlying episcleral vessels are not obscured by the body of the lesion (Grade T1).

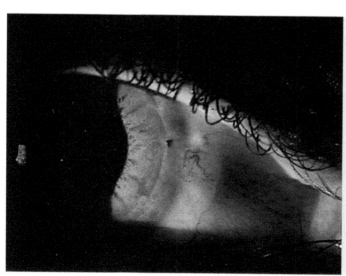

Fig. 2.2 An elevated mound of gelatinous material is seen at the head of this pterygium.

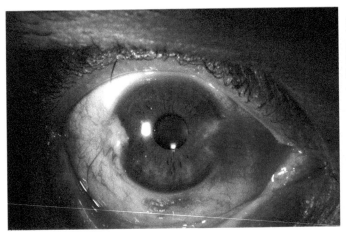

Fig. 2.3 A double-headed pterygium. The nasal lesion is fleshy, red, and progressive (Grade T3), while the temporal one appears less aggressive (Grade T2).

astigmatism. Pterygia typically cause flattening in the horizontal axis and steepening 90 degrees away, that is, they induce with-the-rule astigmatism. The visual impact of pterygia can be assessed by measuring changes in manifest refraction and corneal topography.

2.4 Classification

Though several classification systems have been proposed for pterygium, none has been adopted universally. Here, we will present some of these systems and their underlying rationale.

Pterygia can be graded in terms of the redness of their body[5] as
- Grade I: No redness or faint pinkish hue.
- Grade II: Scattered areas with moderate redness.
- Grade III: Significant diffuse redness.

Alternatively, they can be graded for the vascularity of the body[6] as
- V0: No vascularity.
- V1: Minimal vascularity.
- V2: Normal vascularity.
- V3: Moderate vascularity (denser than conjunctiva) with vessel congestion.
- V4: Severe vascularity with vessel congestion and dilation.

In general, the more red or vascular the pterygium tissue is, the more aggressive it is considered. More vascular pterygia tend to progress fast across the cornea, and they require more aggressive surgical management as they may readily recur.

A different way to grade pterygium lesions has been proposed by Tan et al,[7] and it depends on the fleshiness of the lesion as follows:

- Grade T1: Atrophic pterygium with episcleral vessels not obscured by the body of the lesion (▶ Fig. 2.1).
- Grade T2: Partially obscured episcleral vessels by the body of the lesion (▶ Fig. 2.3 and ▶ Fig. 2.4).
- Grade T3: Fleshy pterygium with episcleral vessels totally obscured by the body of the lesion (▶ Fig. 2.3 and ▶ Fig. 2.5).

In the Tan classification, a fleshier pterygium is thought to be more aggressive.

Regardless of the classification used, the management of white atrophic pterygia should be very different from that of red fleshy ones. Surgical management should be stratified according to the perceived aggressiveness of the lesion on clinical examination. This evaluation of aggressiveness would include the aforementioned characteristics, the age of the patient, continued exposure to risk factors (UV light and irritants), race, possibly gender, and others.[8]

2.5 Differential Diagnosis

The differential diagnosis of pterygium includes
- Fibrovascular pannus.
- OSSN.
- Pseudopterygium secondary to chemical, thermal, or mechanical injury.

Pannus can be seen in any clock hour in the peripheral cornea and is not limited to the 3 or 9 o'clock positions. It does not have a triangular shape, and it is only present within 1 mm from the limbus. Pannus may be caused by chronic contact lens wear, prior trauma to limbal area including surgery, chronic allergies/vernal keratoconjuncti-

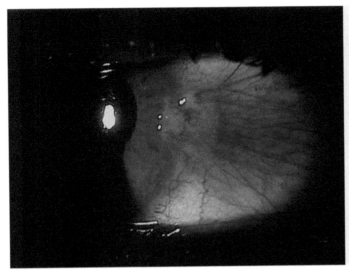

Fig. 2.4 The episcleral vessels are only partially obscured in this Grade T2 pterygium.

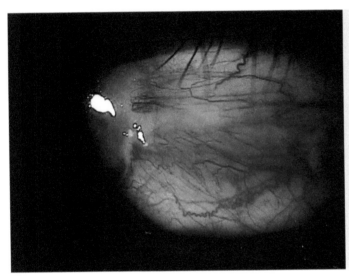

Fig. 2.5 The body of this vascular fleshy pterygium totally obscures the underlying episcleral vessels (Grade T3).

vitis, or meibomian gland disease causing repeated episodes of staphylococcal marginal keratitis. Pannus may be considered the non-inflamed version of a pseudopterygium.

OSSN may also arise from any clock hour at the limbus, though it also has preponderance for the interpalpebral fissure. This is not surprising since exposure to UV radiation is a major risk factor for the development of OSSN. Neoplastic lesions can have a leukoplakic, papillary, gelatinous, or opalescent appearance, and they typically also have feeder vessels. In rare occasions, an OSSN lesion may develop on top of a prior pterygium lesion. In such cases, proper diagnosis can be made with

histologic evaluation of the tissue after excisional biopsy. Alternatively, ultra-high resolution optical coherence tomography may provide an "optical biopsy" of the lesion with thickened hyper-reflective epithelium and an abrupt transition from normal epithelium representing OSSN.

A pseudopterygium develops in cases of significant prior inflammation due to chemical, thermal, or mechanical injury as part of the reparative process that follows such injuries. It is differentiated from a true pterygium by the history of a prior inflammatory insult, its presence in one eye, a location other than the horizontal meridian, and its nonprogressive nature.

2.6 Conclusion

Pterygium is an ocular surface lesion with characteristic wing-shaped appearance at either the 3 or the 9 o'clock position in the palpebral fissure. Atypical pterygia can be differentiated from OSSN lesions either by excisional biopsy or by using the "optical biopsy" that high-resolution optical coherence tomography can provide. There is no unified classification system for pterygium lesions; yet, it is well accepted that more vascular and fleshier lesions tend to be more aggressive and recur after excision.

References

[1] Di Girolamo N, Chui J, Coroneo MT, Wakefield D. Pathogenesis of pterygia: role of cytokines, growth factors, and matrix metalloproteinases. Prog Retin Eye Res. 2004; 23(2):195–228

[2] Chui J, Coroneo MT, Tat LT, Crouch R, Wakefield D, Di Girolamo N. Ophthalmic pterygium: a stem cell disorder with premalignant features. Am J Pathol. 2011; 178(2): 817–827

[3] Kobayashi H, Kohshima S. Unique morphology of the human eye. Nature. 1997; 387(6635):767–768

[4] Coroneo MT, Müller-Stolzenburg NW, Ho A. Peripheral light focusing by the anterior eye and the ophthalmohelioses. Ophthalmic Surg. 1991; 22(12):705–711

[5] Safi H, Kheirkhah A, Mahbod M, Molaei S, Hashemi H, Jabbarvand M. Correlations between histopathologic changes and clinical features in pterygia. J Ophthalmic Vis Res. 2016; 11 (2):153–158

[6] Johnston SC, Williams PB, Sheppard JD. Comprehensive system for pterygium classification. Invest Ophthalmol Vis Sci. 2004; 45:E-abstract:2940

[7] Tan DT, Chee SP, Dear KB, Lim AS. Effect of pterygium morphology on pterygium recurrence in a controlled trial comparing conjunctival autografting with bare sclera excision. Arch Ophthalmol. 1997; 115(10):1235–1240

[8] Donaldson KE, Alfonso EC. Recent advances in pterygium excision. Contemp Ophthalmol. 2003; 2:1–7

3 Current Concepts in Treatments of Pterygium—An Evidence-Based Review

Nathan Rock, Ming Wang, Nancy Argano, and Ilan Cohen

Abstract

This chapter provides an overview of the present evidence with regard to surgical solutions for pterygia. The primary goal of adjunctive surgery techniques is to reduce the recurrence of pterygium. Pertinent literature about conjunctival autograft, pterygium extended removal followed by extended conjunctival transplant, limbal conjunctival allograft (CLAG), and amniotic membrane transplantation are reviewed. Mitomycin C (MMC), 5-fluorouracil (5-FU), and bevacizumab are reviewed as adjunctive agents.

Keywords: pterygium recurrence, conjunctival autograft, tissue adhesive, amniotic membrane, mitomycin C

3.1 Introduction

Pterygia are fibrovascular growths extending from the bulbar conjunctiva onto the cornea. Despite their high prevalence, there is still no consensus regarding the pathophysiology of pterygium formation. Exposure to ultraviolet (UV) radiation is a major risk factor for pterygium formation, but no mechanism has definitively identified which UV light induces the disease. UV exposure is known to cause mutations in the p53 tumor suppressor gene. Studies have linked mutations in the p53 tumor suppressor gene with pterygium formation.[1,2] The corneal limbal epithelium has been suggested to provide a barrier between the conjunctiva and the cornea. Limbal stem cells (LSCs) help maintain a healthy corneal surface by renewing epithelial cells. Pterygia have been proposed to represent a zone of LSC deficiency. Histopathologically, pterygia are characterized by a fragmented Bowman's layer and altered limbal epithelial cells.[1,2]

Surgical excision of a pterygium is indicated when the pterygium approaches the visual axis threatening occlusion or inducing significant irregular astigmatism. Severe irritation, inflammation, restriction of eye movements, or cosmesis can also be surgical indications.[3] The recurrence of pterygium after excision is the primary complication after surgery. Therefore, modern surgical techniques are designed with the primary goal of reducing the recurrence rate of pterygium.

3.2 Defining Recurrence

After excision, pterygium recurrence appears to be related to accelerated fibrovascular proliferation. Recurrence is one of the most commonly encountered postoperative complications. A fibrovascular extension onto the cornea is considered a true corneal recurrence. This is the most common form described in the literature. However, recurrence is sometimes defined in different stages. The most common method to grade recurrence of pterygium is defined by Prabhasawat et al[4] on a 1 to 4 grading scale (▶ Table 3.1).

3.2.1 Current Surgical Management Techniques

Bare Sclera Technique

The first successful management technique for pterygium surgery was introduced in the 1940s. This was the bare sclera technique which involves complete excision of the pterygium head, body, and some of the surrounding normal bulbar conjunctiva including Tenon's capsule. The surrounding normal

Table 3.1 The grades of pterygium recurrence as defined by Prabhasawat et al[4]

Grade 1	Normal appearance of the operated site
Grade 2	Presence of fine episcleral vessels in the excised area, extending to the limbus, but without any fibrous tissue
Grade 3	Presence of fibrovascular tissue in the excised area, reaching the limbus
Grade 4	True corneal recurrence, with fibrovascular tissue invading the cornea

Note that a Grade 4 recurrence is a true corneal recurrence, which is the form most commonly reported by authors.

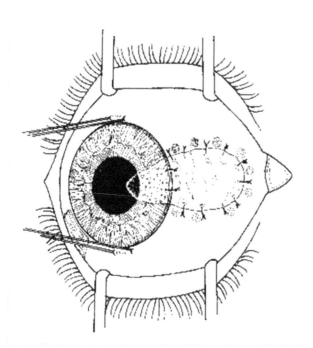

Fig. 3.1 Pterygium surgery with conjunctival allograft secured with sutures. (Reproduced with permission from Tsiouris AJ, Sanelli PC, Comunale JP, eds. Case-Based Brain Imaging. 2nd ed. New York, NY: Thieme; 2013:108.)

bulbar conjunctiva is then sutured to the sclera, leaving a bed of bare sclera next to the corneal limbus.[5]

When primary pterygium excision is completed with the bare sclera technique, the recurrence rate has been reported to be as a high as 24 to 89%.[6] This is likely secondary to compromise to the LSCs in the cornea and lack of coverage of the exposed scleral bed. Because of this high recurrence rate, in modern medicine, this technique is now typically combined with some type of grafting such as a conjunctival or amniotic membrane graft (AMG).

Conjunctival Autograft

Conjunctival Autograft (CAG) involves placement of an autograft over the exposed sclera after pterygium excision. This autograft is generally obtained from the ipsilateral superior bulbar conjunctiva, but can be obtained from the contralateral eye or other quadrants if needed. The preparation is generally made without inclusion of Tenon's capsule.[7] Many surgeons still consider this the first-line approach both for primary and recurrent pterygium. The recurrence rate when CAG is used is 2.6 to 39%.[8] The conjunctival graft can be adhered in several different manners. The most common

include sutures, tissue adhesive, and autologous blood (▶ Fig. 3.1).

Sutures

Sutures are the classical method for adhering the CAG and are still favored by many surgeons. Advantages of sutures are that they are easily available, attained at a low cost, and provide excellent graft stability. Intraoperative issues associated with sutures are that their placement does require more time, which prolongs the total case operating time. Postoperative complications include patient discomfort, possibility of granuloma formation, suture abscesses, giant papillary conjunctivitis, necrosis, and scarring.

Tissue Adhesive

The use of tissue adhesive for adhering the CAG is regarded by some authors as superior to sutures. The two types of fibrin glue most commonly used are the TISSEEL VH fibrin sealant (Baxter) and Evicel (Ethicon).[8] Other preparations include Tissucol Duo Quick (Baxter) and Beriplast P (Aventis).[9] Tissue adhesive preparations are composed of two components: fibrin sealer protein concentrate and thrombin, which are mixed for application. These components are derived from human plasma and are virus inactivated through a treatment process.

Benefits of tissue adhesive include a reduction in surgical time, reduction in postoperative inflammation, and possible reduction in recurrence rate. Graft displacement and graft loss are complications that can occur postoperatively. This can be reduced by ensuring excess glue is removed from the scleral bed intraoperatively. Because of preparation from human plasma, there is a potential risk of transmission of blood-borne diseases. However, preparations are created from a screened donor pool and do go through a viral inactivation process. International safety studies have not shown evidence of transmission of hepatitis virus or human immunodeficiency virus. A risk of allergic reactions has been reported, but the occurrence rate is low at 0.5/100,000 (all reactions) and 0.3/100, 000 (serious reactions). The cost of fibrin adhesive is significantly higher than sutures.[8]

Sutures versus Tissue Adhesive

There have been numerous studies performed directly comparing the efficacy of fibrin glue versus sutures with regard to the recurrence rate. There is a trend that recurrence may be less frequent when fibrin glue is used. For primary pterygium excision with CAG with fibrin glue reported recurrence rates range from to 3.3 to 14%[10,11] and CAG with sutures 8.0 to 20%.[12,13] It is theorized that the reduction in postoperative inflammation is responsible for this. Factors associated with this indicate that less graft manipulation is typically needed intraoperatively when fibrin adhesive is used and that sutures may contribute to mechanical postoperative stress.

Autologous Blood

The use of autologous blood has been used as an alternative method to adhere the conjunctival graft. In this technique, the bare sclera is allowed to bleed for several minutes until a small film forms. The free graft is then held in firm apposition to the scleral bed for 6 to 7 minutes.[9,14] The graft is checked for stability after surgery, and a pressure patch is applied until postoperative day 1. Benefits of this procedure are that it uses the patient's own clotting factors, which avoids any chance of allergic or immune response to fibrin adhesives. Drawbacks include increased operating times and risk of graft dehiscence or loss as the

adherence can be less pronounced than traditional adhesive.

As this technique is a relatively newer application, and there are fewer trials evaluating its success, a study of 10 patients by Xu et al[9] with this technique indicates recurrence rate comparable to that of fibrin adhesive (10%) with no cases of graft dehiscence, which leads the authors to recommend its use. A larger trial of 62 eyes by Nadarajah et al[14] with this technique did show a similar recurrence rate (10.6%), but a significant risk of graft dehiscence (24.2%), which leads the authors to express caution about its use. Surgeon-dependent factors are likely responsible for this difference, but further study on this technique is needed.

3.2.2 Pterygium-Extended Removal Followed by Extended Conjunctival Transplant

Pterygium Extended Removal Followed by Extended Conjunctival Transplant (PERFECT) is a variation of conjunctival allograft. In this technique, a significantly larger portion of the surrounding conjunctiva is excised surrounding the pterygium, and a corresponding large graft is dissected and placed. Subconjunctival Tenon's fascia dissection is completed from the limbus to 10 to 15 mm posterior to the limbus. The dissection extends approximately 2 clock hours above and below the conjunctival wound margins almost to the superior and inferior rectus muscles. A corresponding area of superior bulbar conjunctiva is excised to Tenon's capsule. The large graft is placed and sutured to the bare sclera bed.

The recurrence rate for this technique is reported between 0 and 1.6%. The low recurrence rate is the primary benefit of the procedure. Intraoperative drawbacks include longer operating times, the need for peribulbar or retrobulbar anesthesia, and increased surgical trauma. There is also risk for donor-site complications due to the large size of conjunctival graft that is needed. Transient diplopia has also been reported due to the close proximity to the extraocular muscles encountered during the surgery.[15]

Hirst reported a series of 1,000 patients who had excision with PERFECT. All patients completed at least 1 year of follow-up. A recurrence was observed in only 0.1% of patients. Complication rates were low, but included strabismus, inclusion cyst, granuloma, and a corneal ulcer.[16]

3.2.3 Limbal Conjunctival Allograft

Limbal conjunctival allograft (CLAG) is a variant of conjunctival allograft that involves dissection and inclusion of a portion of the corneal limbus in the graft. The pterygium is excised in the usual manner. The conjunctival graft is created with a length matching the limbal defect with inclusion of clear cornea between 0.5 and 1.0 mm.[3,17] The graft is then translocated to the recipient bed and is secured with either sutures or tissue adhesive.

This technique has been shown to have a reduced recurrence rate versus a free conjunctival flap with rates ranging from 0 to 14.6%.[3,18] It is hypothesized that the inclusion of LSCs acts as a barrier to recurrence. The low recurrence rate is a benefit of this procedure. Drawbacks include increased operating time and potential for donor-site complications.

Masters and Harris reported a large retrospective study of 234 procedures with CLAG with a median follow-up of 25.5 months. A 0.5 mm of clear cornea was included in the conjunctival graft, which was adhered with sutures. Recurrences were observed in 2.14% of patients overall with recurrence in 0.57% of eyes with primary pterygium and 6.9% cases with recurrent pterygium.[3]

3.2.4 Amniotic Membrane Graft

AMG have been described considerably for the treatment of pterygium. AMG are used for their anti-inflammatory, anti-scarring, and anti-angiogenic properties. AMG are either cryopreserved or dehydrated. For pterygium surgery, the pterygium is excised in the usual manner, and an amniotic membrane is applied over the exposed scleral bed, generally with fibrin glue.[19] The recurrence rate for these procedures has been demonstrated between 0 and 40.9%[20,21,22] (▶ Fig. 3.2).

There have been numerous trials that compare outcomes for patients who receive CAG compared to those who receive amniotic membrane transplantation (AMT). The majority of the trials demonstrate a lower recurrence rate for patients who receive CAG versus AMT. The range of recurrence in these trials ranges between 4.76 and 16% for conjunctival autografts and 11.1 and 40.9% with AMT.[22,23,24,25,26] In contrast, Küçükerdönmez et al report results in a randomized trial, which do show similar results between CAG and AMT for both primary and recurrent pterygium. In this study with CAG, recurrence is reported at 7.5% and AMT at 7.9%.[27] A large Cochrane Review meta-analysis included 1947 eyes that had undergone either CAG or AMT. The review indicated that

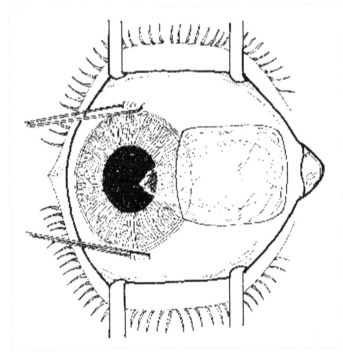

Fig. 3.2 "Pterygium surgery with amniotic membrane graft secured with tissue adhesive." (Reproduced with permission from Hersh P, Zagelbaum B, Cremers S. Ophthalmic Surgical Procedures. 2nd ed. New York, NY: Thieme; 2009:108.)

there was a lower risk of recurrence for patients who had undergone CAG versus AMT.[28]

Because there is a trend of higher recurrence with AMG versus CAG, some authors do report that they reserve AMG after pterygium surgery in circumstances when grafting procedures are contraindicated. This could include cases when preexisting conjunctival scarring makes harvesting of a donor conjunctival graft difficult or cases for very large or double-headed pterygia. It is also preferred for glaucoma patients where the superior conjunctiva must be left intact for a filtration bleb.[19]

3.3 Adjunctive Agents

There are several agents that can be applied with a goal of reduction of pterygium recurrence. These agents can be used preoperatively, intraoperatively, or postoperatively. Preoperative use involves subconjunctival injection prior to surgery. The most common method of use is intraoperatively. Intraoperatively, the agents are typically applied to the exposed scleral bed and then rinsed. Postoperative use can include topical application by the patient in the form of compounded drops or subconjunctival injection by the surgeon if a recurrence appears imminent. The most common agents are mitomycin C (MMC), 5-fluorouracil (5-FU), and bevacizumab.[29] Most trials have compared the use of these adjunctive agents compared to bare sclera excision. An increasing area of research is in the combination an adjunctive surgery, such as CAG or AMT, with an adjunctive agent. This is a promising area of research, but there is currently not enough evidence in this area to draw strong conclusions.[30]

3.3.1 Mitomycin C

MMC is an antibiotic-antineoplastic compound that works as an alkylating agent that selectively inhibits deoxyribonucleic acid (DNA) replication, mitosis, and protein synthesis. This results in antiproliferative effects on fibroblasts and vascular endothelial cells. The use of MMC has been extensively described for pterygium excision. While generally well tolerated, it can result in significant and visually threatening complications, including scleral thinning, scleral melts, cataract formation, loss of best-corrected visual acuity, iritis, and spontaneous postoperative globe perforation.

Intraoperatively, it can be applied in concentrations ranging from 0.02 to 0.04% and is generally

used for 3 to 5 minutes. Numerous trials have been completed to evaluate the use of MMC, and they are nearly universal in showing statistically significant reduction in pterygium reccurrence versus bare sclera excision. Several studies have also evaluated the use of 0.02 to 0.04% topical MMC applied postoperatively two times a day (BID) to four times a day (QID). Data from these trials also support a reduction in reccurrence versus bare sclera excision and compare favorably to the rate of intraoperative application. However, due to the risk of significant complications, most surgeons advocate for its use only in a controlled intraoperative setting versus applied topically postoperatively.[30]

A novel study by Kareem et al recruited patients with primary bilateral pterygium and treated a cohort of patients with one eye with bare sclera excision and one eye with excision and 0.5 mg/mL MMC. The recurrence rate was 8% for eyes treated with MMC and 32% for fellow eyes. No adverse events were encountered.[31]

3.3.2 5-Fluorouracil

5-FU is a pyrimidine analog that inhibits DNA synthesis. 5-FU is known to be less potent then MMC as it works only on fibroblasts. The side effect profile is the same as MMC and includes scleral thinning, scleral melts, cataract formation, and loss of best-corrected visual acuity, iritis, and spontaneous postoperative globe perforation.[31]

The previously described study by Kareem et al for patients with primary bilateral pterygium also treated cohort of patients with one eye with bare sclera excision and one eye with excision and 50 mg/mL MMC. The recurrence rate was 18% for eyes treated with MMC and 34% for fellow eyes. No adverse events were encountered. While the recurrence rate was acceptably low, the authors note that the cosmetic results were less satisfactory than MMC as 5-FU resulted in more abnormal conjunctival vasculature.[31]

3.3.3 Bevacizumab

Bevacizumab (Avastin) is an anti-VEGF antibody. Bevacizumab prevents the interaction between VEGF-A and its receptor on endothelial cells. This blocks the signal pathway leading to endothelial cell proliferation and new blood vessel formation. Bevacizumab is typically applied intraoperatively via subconjunctival injection though its use has been reported postoperatively as an injection or topical drops.[32] In contrast to antimetabolites, no serious adverse events have been reported with bevacizumab for use in pterygium excision.[33]

However, compared to other adjunctive agents, there is mixed evidence regarding the efficacy of the agent. A large 2014 meta-analysis by Hu et al included 482 eyes from 9 randomized clinical trials of patients with pterygium treated with bevacizumab. The analysis confirms that the treatment is safe, but it did indicate there was no statistically significant reduction in recurrence.

3.4 Conclusion

A review of the recent literature on pterygium is generally universal in recommendation that some form of adjunctive surgery or agent should be used versus bare sclera excision with the goal of reducing the recurrence of pterygium. There is a trend that recurrence may be the lowest with PERFECT and CLAG. These procedures are more technically complicated and generally require longer operating times. Low recurrence is also observed with conjunctival allografts, which trend to show slightly more efficacy versus AMG. In general, there is trend that the most affective adjective agent is MMC. However, some authors reserve adjunctive agents, such as MMC, for recurrent pterygium surgeries only due to the additional risks.

Despite trends in the literature, we understand that each surgeon will have protocols that can provide results that exceed those reported in trials. This book details the best practices for many of these techniques. There are many variations, such as graft size, use of glue versus sutures, concentration of adjunctive agents, and other variables, that can significantly affect outcomes. For instance, Ilan Cohen, MD, reports a technique that reduces the operating time of CLAG to a level similar to traditional grafting techniques. A forthcoming retrospective review of this procedure includes 25 eyes of primary pterygium and indicates a 0% recurrence rate.

The modified CLAG approach is performed under topical anesthesia. Topical tetracaine is applied to the eye on a Weck-Cel sponge focusing on the pterygium for at least 1 minute prior to dissection. The area and the extent of the pterygium are marked using a marking pen. Eraser wet field cautery is applied to a small point on the line to initiate an incision using Westcott scissors without causing a significant hemorrhage. The scissors are used to spread the entire area under the pterygium including Tenon's capsule to the greatest extent possible. Lidocaine is applied gently using a 27G blunt irrigation cannula under the conjunctiva with care taken not to cause significant inflation of Tenon's capsule.

Hot, handheld cautery is applied to the edges of the pterygium to cut it away from the conjunctiva. Eraser cautery is used as needed on the specific points of bleeding on the sclera while making sure not to completely ablate conjunctival vessels that are needed to feed the graft. The control of bleeding during the surgery is essential for the reduction of surgical time and optimizing the surgical view.

The pterygium is gently peeled away from the limbus anteriorly using a blunt instrument to help the separation. Care must be taken not to cut too deeply into the corneal stroma in this process even if it contains some pterygium fibers that penetrated deep.

A burr is used to smooth the area of the cornea where the pterygium was removed. Attention is directed to the superior conjunctiva and the patient is asked to look down as far as possible. The area of the conjunctiva to be excised is marked, while the limbus remains unmarked to help with orientation. The conjunctiva is also marked with an "S" to prevent possible inversion and for orientation. The graft area is cut with Wescott scissors while taking care to obtain conjunctiva with as little Tenon's as possible. The spreading of conjunctiva is achieved by using dull point Wescott scissors. Eraser Cautery is used as needed in this stage. The graft is reflected back on the cornea near the limbus and a crescent blade is used to gently dissect under the conjunctiva reaching anteriorly into cornea about 0.75 to 1.00 mm from the limbus at about 75 to 100-µm depth. The whole conjunctiva-LSC complex is cut away using fine scissors or a blade.

This complex is now brought on to the pterygium site while making sure that the limbal edge is aligned and attached to limbus at the same distance away from the limbus as it was cut from the donor site. The conjunctiva is laid flat on the sclera. There is no need to attempt any tucking, and it is normal at this stage to have a small exposed area of sclera between the graft and the remaining conjunctival edges. Care must be taken to ensure that the graft is right side up and not tucked underneath itself.

TISSEEL tissue glue is applied using two pierce cannulas at each syringe in the following manner: The first glue component (blue) is applied, while the pierce cannula is sliding gently under the graft making sure that there is a thin layer underneath the graft. The second component (black) is then applied in a similar fashion although in much less quantity. Then the two pierce cannulas are used to wipe the surface of the graft to spread the glue and express any excess, while the graft is stuck in place. Any excess glue is cut away from the eye using scissors in order to prevent tissue entanglement. The patient receives topical antibiotic and steroid and is then patched.

References

[1] Chui J, Coroneo MT, Tat LT, Crouch R, Wakefield D, Di Girolamo N. Ophthalmic pterygium: a stem cell disorder with premalignant features. Am J Pathol. 2011; 178(2):817–827

[2] Dushku N, John MK, Schultz GS, Reid TW. Pterygia pathogenesis: corneal invasion by matrix metalloproteinase expressing altered limbal epithelial basal cells. Arch Ophthalmol. 2001; 119(5):695–706

[3] Masters JS, Harris DJ , Jr. Low recurrence rate of pterygium after excision with conjunctival limbal autograft: a retrospective study with long-term follow-up. Cornea. 2015; 34(12):1569–1572

[4] Prabhasawat P, Barton K, Burkett G, Tseng SC. Comparison of conjunctival autografts, amniotic membrane grafts, and primary closure for pterygium excision. Ophthalmology. 1997; 104(6):974–985

[5] Sheppard JD, Mansur A, Comstock TL, Hovanesian JA. An update on the surgical management of pterygium and the role of loteprednol etabonate ointment. Clin Ophthalmol. 2014; 8:1105–1118

[6] Jaros PA, DeLuise VP. Pingueculae and pterygia. Surv Ophthalmol. 1988; 33(1):41–49

[7] Prajna NV, Devi L, Seeniraj SK, Keenan JD. Conjunctival autograft versus amniotic membrane transplantation after double pterygium excision: a randomized trial. Cornea. 2016; 35(6):823–826

[8] Ratnalingam V, Eu ALK, Ng GL, Taharin R, John E. Fibrin adhesive is better than sutures in pterygium surgery. Cornea. 2010; 29(5):485–489

[9] Xu F, Li M, Yan Y, Lu K, Cui L, Chen Q. A novel technique of sutureless and glueless conjunctival autografting in pterygium surgery by electrocautery pen. Cornea. 2013; 32(3):290–295

[10] Koranyi G, Seregard S, Kopp ED. Cut and paste: a no suture, small incision approach to pterygium surgery. Br J Ophthalmol. 2004; 88(7):911–914

[11] Syam PP, Eleftheriadis H, Liu CSC. Inferior conjunctival autograft for primary pterygia. Ophthalmology. 2003; 110(4):806–810

[12] Farid M, Pirnazar JR. Pterygium recurrence after excision with conjunctival autograft: a comparison of fibrin tissue adhesive to absorbable sutures. Cornea. 2009; 28(1):43–45

[13] Elwan SAM. Comparison between sutureless and glue free versus sutured limbal conjunctival autograft in primary pterygium surgery. Saudi J Ophthalmol. 2014; 28(4):292–298

[14] Nadarajah G, Ratnalingam VH, Isa HM. Autologous blood versus fibrin glue in pterygium excision. Cornea. 2016(Dec):1–5

[15] Cornelius CR. Recurrence rate and complications of pterygium extended removal followed by extended conjunctival transplant. Cornea. 2017; 36(1):101–103

[16] Hirst LW. Recurrence and complications after 1,000 surgeries using pterygium extended removal followed by extended conjunctival transplant. Ophthalmology. 2012; 119(11):2205–2210

[17] Patel D, Vala R, Shah H, et al. Efficacy of limbal conjunctival autograft surgery with stem cells in primary and recurrent pterygium. Gujarat Med J.. 2015; 70(1):17–20

[18] Mutlu FM, Sobaci G, Tatar T, Yildirim E. A comparative study of recurrent pterygium surgery: limbal conjunctival autograft transplantation versus mitomycin C with conjunctival flap. Ophthalmology. 1999; 106(4):817–821

[19] Noureddin GS, Yeung SN. The use of dry amniotic membrane in pterygium surgery. Clin Ophthalmol. 2016; 10:705–712

[20] Jain AK, Bansal R, Sukhija J. Human amniotic membrane transplantation with fibrin glue in management of primary pterygia: a new tuck-in technique. Cornea. 2008; 27(1):94–99

[21] Fernandes M, Sangwan VS, Bansal AK, et al. Outcome of pterygium surgery: analysis over 14 years. Eye (Lond). 2005; 19(11):1182–1190

[22] Tananuvat N, Martin T. The results of amniotic membrane transplantation for primary pterygium compared with conjunctival autograft. Cornea. 2004; 23(5):458–463

[23] Özer A, Yildirim N, Erol N, Yurdakul S. Long-term results of bare sclera, limbal-conjunctival autograft and amniotic membrane graft techniques in primary pterygium excisions. Ophthalmologica. 2009; 223(4):269–273

[24] Luanratanakorn P, Ratanapakorn T, Suwan-Apichon O, Chuck RS. Randomised controlled study of conjunctival autograft versus amniotic membrane graft in pterygium excision. Br J Ophthalmol. 2006; 90(12):1476–1480

[25] Katircioğlu YA, Altiparmak UE, Duman S. Comparison of three methods for the treatment of pterygium: amniotic membrane graft, conjunctival autograft and conjunctival autograft plus mitomycin C. Orbit. 2007; 26(1):5–13

[26] Toker E, Eraslan M. Recurrence after primary pterygium excision: amniotic membrane transplantation with fibrin glue versus conjunctival autograft with fibrin glue. Curr Eye Res. 2016; 41(1):1–8

[27] Küçükerdönmez C, Akova YA, Altinörs DD. Comparison of conjunctival autograft with amniotic membrane transplantation for pterygium surgery: surgical and cosmetic outcome. Cornea. 2007; 26(4):407–413

[28] Clearfield E, Muthappan V, Wang X, Kuo IC. Conjunctival autograft for pterygium. Cochrane Database Syst Rev. 2016; 2 (2):CD011349

[29] Alsmman AH, Radwan G, Abozaid MA, Mohammed UA, Abd Elhaleim NG. Preoperative subconjunctival combined injection of bevacizumab and mitomycin C before the surgical excision of primary pterygium: clinical and histological results. Clin Ophthalmol. 2017; 11:493–501

[30] Kaufman SC, Jacobs DS, Lee WB, Deng SX, Rosenblatt MI, Shtein RM. Options and adjuvants in surgery for pterygium: a report by the American Academy of Ophthalmology. Ophthalmology. 2013; 120(1):201–208

[31] Kareem AA, Farhood QK, Alhammami HA. The use of antimetabolites as adjunctive therapy in the surgical treatment of pterygium. Clin Ophthalmol. 2012; 6(1):1849–1854

[32] Shenasi A, Mousavi F, Shoa-Ahari S, Rahimi-Ardabili B, Fouladi RF. Subconjunctival bevacizumab immediately after excision of primary pterygium: the first clinical trial. Cornea. 2011; 30(11):1219–1222

[33] Enkvetchakul O, Thanathanee O, Rangsin R, Lekhanont K, Suwan-Apichon O. A randomized controlled trial of intralesional bevacizumab injection on primary pterygium: preliminary results. Cornea. 2011; 30(11):1213–1218

4 Evolution of the Medical and Surgical Treatments for Pterygium

Ahmed A. Abdelghany and Jorge L. Alio

Abstract

Pterygium is a non-malignant slow-growing proliferation of wing-shaped fibrovascular tissue, thought to originate from limbal stem cells altered by chronic ultraviolet (UV) exposure. It arises from subconjunctival tissue and may extend over the cornea thus disturbing the vision. It is seen more frequently in tropical and subtropical areas where exposure to UV sunlight is high. Pterygium causes cosmetic imbalance of the ocular surface with chronic hyperemia and frequent discomfort in the affected patients; it is frequently progressive toward the cornea being potentially the source of optical changes in the anterior corneal surface, such as progressive astigmatism and higher order aberrations. For all these reasons, it frequently requires surgical excision. The main aim of pterygium surgery is to eliminate it, prevent its recurrence, and restore the ocular surface integrity and cosmetics. In our chapter, we are going to discuss different techniques for pterygium management.

Keywords: pterygium, recurrent pterygium, limbal autograft, mitomycin C

4.1 Introduction

Pterygium was first described in 1000 BC by Sushruta, the first ophthalmic surgeon according to the literature.[1]

Over the years, many medical treatments involving bile, urine, acids, radiotherapy, thiotepa, 5-fluorouracil, and mitomycin C (MMC) have been used. In the past, the use of horsehair was described to remove pterygium.[2]

Surgery is indicated when the patient is feeling discomfort despite lubricant eye drops, when there is restriction of ocular motility, growth on the visual axis, and aesthetic complaints.[3]

There are many approaches described for the surgical removal of pterygium. The most common surgical techniques include excision of the conjunctiva and the proliferated fibrotic subconjunctival tissue, leaving the bare sclera, using a conjunctival or conjunctival limbal autograft, coverage of the excised area with amniotic membrane (AM) or the use of antiproliferative and antifibrotic adjuncts, such as MMC.[4]

The main aim of pterygium surgery is to eliminate it, prevent its recurrence, and restore the ocular surface integrity and cosmetics.

In this chapter, we will review different modalities of treatments used for pterygium (▶ Table 4.1).

4.2 Simple Excision with Bare Sclera

Simple excision was the first surgical treatment prescribed for pterygium leaving bare sclera, but was associated with high recurrence rate ranging from 40 to 70%.[5,6] It was first described in 1948.[7]

To prevent recurrence, adjunctive therapies are to be considered. These include application of antimetabolites, such as MMC, radiotherapy, conjunctival or limbal conjunctival autograft,[8] and AM graft.

4.3 Simple Excision with Primary Closure

Primary closure is a technique that involves excision of the pterygium, followed by suturing of the remaining conjunctiva on either side of the wound over the bare sclera, to close the defect. This procedure has also been reported to have an unacceptably high rate of recurrence (45–70%) compared to newer techniques.[9]

4.4 Mitomycin C

MMC is an alkylating agent, which inhibits deoxyribonucleic acid (DNA) synthesis. By inhibiting DNA synthesis, it leads to the death of cells caused by the inability to repair the genotoxic injury due to alkylation. It acts against all cells regardless of the cell cycle and even acts in cells that are not synthesizing DNA. Inhibition of DNA synthesis leads to reduction in the number of mitoses, especially when MMC comes into contact with cells that are in the late G1 and early S phases of the cell cycle.

Table 4.1 Different techniques for pterygium surgery

Technique	Advantages	Disadvantages	Authors' personal experience
Simple excision with bare sclera	Easy	High recurrence rate	We do not perform this technique due to high rate of recurrence
Simple excision with primary closure	Easy Less postoperative pain compared to first technique	High recurrence rate	We don't perform this technique due to high rate of recurrence
Mitomycin C	Decreased recurrence rate	Higher concentrations have many complications	Mitomycin C 0.02% is effective with minimal complications
Cyclosporine	Reported to decrease recurrence rate	Many complications	No role in pterygium surgery
Bevacizumab	Reported to decrease recurrence rate	Not effective for preventing recurrence	Inhibit fibrovascular tissue proliferation more than decreasing recurrence rate
β-Irradiation	Reported to decrease recurrence rate	Significant complications	Abandoned nowadays due to problems in its availability and teratogenicity
Conjunctival autograft and limbal conjunctival autograft	Decreased recurrence rate Good cosmetic appearance	Time consuming Interfere with glaucoma surgery if needed later	Good and effective technique with satisfying results
Amniotic membrane grafting	Decreased recurrence rate	If fresh, may transmit infection Difficult preservation in developing world	Results of this technique are not encouraging
Mini-SLET	Decreased recurrence rate	Time consuming	Recommended if autograft is not possible
Tailored corneo-conjunctival autografting	Has lowest recurrence rate reported	Time consuming	Lowest recurrence rate reported No major complications Better cosmetic appearance
Subconjunctival excision	More anatomical excision (the conjunctiva is not involved in pterygium but the Tenon's capsule) Better wound healing, less scarring, and less recurrence rate	No long-term studies	Low recurrence rate Better wound healing and less scarring Fast surgery Minimally invasive

Abbreviation: Mini-SLET, minor ipsilateral simple limbal epithelial transplantation.

It can be used before, during, or after pterygium surgery by applying locally or in the form of eye drops. The injection application directly on the pterygium has the advantage of protecting the corneal endothelium and epithelium. Subconjunctival injection allows a more precise dose to be applied to the patient's eye, which usually does not occur with MMC application while using sponges directly on the sclera during surgery. Its action in the prevention of pterygium recurrence occurs by inhibition of fibroblast proliferation in the episcleral region.

The increased concentration and duration of the application may be associated with complications such as necrotizing scleritis, scleral calcification, ulceration, corneal edema, iritis, glaucoma, cataract, hypotony by injury of the ciliary body, and damage to the corneal epithelium and endothelium.[10,11,12]

The administration of MMC in the pterygium surgery is considered off-label by the Food and Drug Administration (FDA), but it is used in cancer treatment.

4.4.1 Mitomycin C during the Surgery

Twenty-two trials[9,13,14,15,16,17,18,19,20,21,22,23,24,25,26,27,28,29,30,31,32,33] that used MMC in different concentrations (0.002–0.4% for 3–5 min) applied to the bare sclera after pterygium excision were evaluated. Some studies with primary pterygium determined that all MMC concentrations, from 0.002 to 0.04%, given for 3 to 5 minutes, significantly reduced (< 0.0045) the recurrence of pterygium when compared to excision with bare sclera.[9,14,16,19]

The recurrence rate reported in the literature for intraoperative use of MMC in primary pterygium surgery varies from 6.7 to 22.5%.[33,34] The most common dose, according to the literature, is 0.02% for 3 minutes in the bare sclera.[35]

Complications related to the intraoperative use of MMC vary according to the concentration and the duration of application. With the most commonly used dose of 0.02% for 3 minutes, there were no severe complications reported.[35]

Delayed epithelialization can occur with the use of intraoperative MMC 0.04% for 3 to 5 minutes, but it was not reported with MMC 0.02% for 3 minutes. Iritis and corneal dellen have been reported in 3% of cases when MMC 0.01% was used for 5 minutes intraoperatively.[14]

4.4.2 Mitomycin C after the Surgery

The analysis included 12 trials[17,18,19,23,26,27,28,29,32,36,37,38] with application of different concentrations of MMC after surgery at different times. In two studies with MMC application postoperatively (0.02% twice a day for 5 days), there was reduced primary pterygium recurrence.[23,26] High concentrations of MMC (0.04%, 3 to 4 times daily for 7 days) result in a significant reduction in the recurrence of pterygium compared to excision with bare sclera.[38] Studies with primary pterygium[24,27] or combined with recurrent pterygium[26,28] reported no significant changes, comparing the intraoperative or postoperative use of MMC. Sclera ulceration occurred in a proportion that varied from 5 to 19% in eyes with postoperative MMC 0.02% applied twice daily for 5 days,[17] with MMC 0.02% applied 4 times daily for 7 days[24] and 0.04% applied 3 times daily for 7 days.[28] Iritis and corneal dellen occurred with postoperative use of MMC 0.02% 4 times daily for 7 days in 3% of the cases.[28] Two studies[14,18]

have shown increased risk of scleral thinning with increasing concentration of MMC application.

4.4.3 Mitomycin C before the Surgery

The preoperative subconjunctival injection of MMC, in a study of 25 eyes, proved to be efficient, with two cases of delayed epithelialization. Ninety-two percent of eyes with MMC application experienced no recurrence, and 8% had a 2-week delay in corneal epithelialization. No serious complications were reported.[39] Donnenfeld et al reported the efficiency and safety of using preoperative MMC injection of 0.1 mL (0.15 mg/mL) in the pterygium body 1 month prior to the surgery for pterygium recurrence. The results showed less vascularization and inflammation within the pterygium 1 month after injection of MMC with a 6% recurrence after 2 years of follow-up.[40]

The risk of preoperative injection is due to the impossibility of washing the MMC that is in the subconjunctival space and can generate toxicity. Studies showed that subconjunctival injection of MMC 0.2 mL (0.4 mg/mL) injected 2 mm posterior to the limbus caused cell changes, such as flattening and pyknotic nuclei in the ciliary body epithelium, leading to reduction of aqueous humor production a month after the injection.[41]

Our personal results with this technique are very good without reported complications. We use MMC preoperatively in the preparation of surgery for reoperations. Four weeks before the surgery, we inject 0.2 cc of MMC, 0.02% subconjunctivally. Then the surgery is performed as usual (we only perform subconjunctival excision of the pterygium respecting the conjunctiva and without conjunctival flap transposition). In over 100 cases, we have not observed any complication, and our recurrence rate is 2%. This technique is time saving and is very effective in our hands.

4.5 Cyclosporine

Cyclosporine is an immunosuppressant that selectively suppresses T-helper cells, controls interleukin synthesis and secretion, and inhibits vascular endothelial growth factor (VEGF).[42]

Topical cyclosporine is relatively effective in inhibiting pterygium recurrence, but topical cyclosporine causes minor complications, such as irritation, hyperemia, and rarely, scleromalacia.[43]

Turan-Vural et al[44] divided 36 eyes (34 patients) with primary pterygium into two groups and reported that the rate of recurrence was 44.4% in the group that received pterygium surgery using the bare sclera method alone, but was 22.2% in the group receiving postoperative instillation of 0.05% cyclosporine.

The cyclosporine-treated group showed no adverse reaction other than a mild burning sensation and irritation upon application.

For 31 patients (62 eyes) diagnosed with bilateral pterygium, Yalcin Tok et al[45] instilled 0.05% cyclosporine in the right eye, using the left eye as a control, and reported a rate of recurrence of 12.9% in the right eye and 45.2% in the left eye, which indicated that cyclosporine was effective in reducing pterygium recurrence.

Nowadays, there is no role of cyclosporine in pterygium surgery.

4.6 Bevacizumab

Bevacizumab is an anti-VEGF antibody that inhibits angiogenesis and has been studied as an adjuvant therapy to inhibit post-surgery pterygium recurrence.[46] Bevacizumab, a recombinant human monoclonal antibody, is an inhibitor that binds to all biologically active forms of VEGF. In 2004, the FDA approved the drug for the treatment of metastatic colorectal cancer.

In addition, bevacizumab showed promising results in ophthalmology for the treatment of many diseases related to angiogenesis, such as macular degeneration-related choroidal neovascularization, proliferative diabetic retinopathy, and retinal vein occlusion.[47,48]

Bevacizumab can cause severe systemic problems, such as endophthalmitis and arterial thromboembolic events.[49,50]

Motarjemizadeh et al[51] enrolled 90 patients (90 eyes) who underwent pterygium excision and categorized them into three groups. At 24 hours after surgery, group II and group III received a 5 and 10 mg/mL dose of topical bevacizumab, respectively, whereas patients in group I were administered only a placebo starting 1 day after surgery. Participants were instructed to instill their topical medicines four times a day for 1 week. These authors concluded that 10 mg/mL of topical bevacizumab was more efficacious than 5 mg/mL in preventing pterygium recurrence. Ozgurhan et al[46] divided 44 patients (44 eyes) who underwent excision of recurrent pterygium with conjunctival autograft into two groups, one of which was instilled with bevacizumab four times a day for a month, starting 1 month after surgery. Bevacizumab failed to reduce recurrence, but effectively inhibited angiogenesis.

Suh and Choi[52] divided 54 patients (54 eyes) who underwent primary pterygium surgical excision into two groups and, after administering subconjunctival bevacizumab injections to one group, reported that it failed to affect recurrence, but successfully inhibited proliferation of fibrovascular tissues.

4.7 β-Irradiation

β-irradiation has also been found to be a relatively well-tolerated procedure, with recurrence rates similar to chemotherapeutic agents and conjunctival autografting. Rare but significant complications of this procedure include scleral thinning, ulceration, infection, and radiation-induced cataract.[53] This type of therapy is abandoned nowadays due to problems in its availability and teratogenicity.

4.8 Conjunctival Autograft and Limbal Conjunctival Autograft

In conjunctival autograft surgery, conjunctival tissue from another part of the person's eye along with limbal tissue is resected in one piece and is used to cover the area from which the pterygium was excised.

There is widespread acceptance of conjunctival autografting and application to pterygium by Vastine et al and Kenyon et al.[8] However, no single autograft technique is completely effective in preventing recurrence. Pterygium excision followed by conjunctival autograft is associated with recurrence rate of 5.3 to 39%.[8]

After the initial report by Kenyon et al, describing the success of conjunctival autografting following pterygium excision, other authors have largely failed to achieve the same success rate.[6,8] The wide range of recurrence rates reported number of factors. Review of published literature suggests that the surgical technique could probably be the single most important factor influencing recurrence. The meticulousness with which the limbal tissue is included in the autograft, in our opinion, determines the success of the procedure. Various studies have specifically described the inclusion of limbal tissue in the graft and have demonstrated low recurrence rates.[8,54]

Limbal autografts have been used successfully to correct limbal dysfunction, acting as a barrier against conjunctival invasion of the cornea and supplying stem cells of the corneal epithelium.

The importance of limbal transplantation in ensuring low recurrence rates has also been stressed by Figueiredo et al.[55] A major drawback for limbal conjunctival autograft transplantation is that it is technically more demanding and time consuming.

4.8.1 Amniotic Membrane Grafting

AM being a basement membrane acts as a new healthy substrate suitable for proper epithelization. It has a strong anti-adhesive effect[56] being normally avascular and thus it inhibits the incursion of new vessels.[57]

AM grafts are thought to promote healing and reduce rates of recurrence because of their anti-inflammatory properties, their promotion of epithelial growth, and their suppression of transforming growth factor β (TGF- β) signaling and fibroblast proliferation.[9]

In the 1940s, AM use in the treatment of ocular surface conditions was described.[57] Since 1995, it has been increasingly used to treat a variety of ocular surface conditions,[58] including persistent corneal epithelial defects, acute chemical burns, and cicatrizing conditions, such as Stevens–Johnson syndrome and ocular cicatricial pemphigoid.[58] Amniotic membrane transplantation (AMT) has been used in the reconstruction of fornices, as a covering following excision of conjunctival lesions, and in limbal stem cell deficiency with concomitant limbal stem cell grafting.[58]

AM can be prepared fresh or preserved using either freeze-drying of the membrane (dry AM) or cryopreservation. Fresh AM is more commonly used in the developing world, where preservation techniques are not easily performed.[59] Unfortunately, the use of fresh AM is less advantageous, not only because it must be used in a limited time and does not exploit the size of the membrane for multiple tissue transplantations, but it also poses a greater risk of transmitting infection.[59]

Cryopreservation of AM is achieved by freezing fresh AM in either phosphate-buffered saline in dimethyl sulfoxide or in Eagle's Minimum Essential Medium (MEM) with glycerol, both at –80 °C.[59]

Recurrence rates of pterygia following amniotic membrane grafting (AMG) are cited between 14.5 and 27.3%.[9]

Reported complications include wound dehiscence, Tenon's granuloma, conjunctival cysts, necrotizing scleritis, and subconjunctival fibrosis from the donor site.[60]

Our personal experience with this technique is not good and results were not encouraging.

4.8.2 Minor Ipsilateral Simple Limbal Epithelial Transplantation

AM graft to cover the bare sclera area is combined with a small autologous simple limbal epithelial transplant (mini-SLET) to provide stem cells at the limbal area.[61] Mini-SLET is recommended for pterygium in cases that are not good candidates for a conjunctival autograft.

4.8.3 Tailored Corneo-Conjunctival Autografting

A tailored corneo-conjunctival graft was prepared from the superior side with the same size of the bared sclera sparing the deep Tenon at the donor bed in the conjunctival part for rapid spontaneous healing without scar, and a crescent knife was used to dissect about 3 mm from the upper cornea with nearly the same thickness as conjunctiva to be included in the graft[62] (► Fig. 4.1). Tailored corneo-conjunctival graft offers the advantage of preventing recurrence in addition to better cosmetic appearance of the tailored graft (► Fig. 4.2).

This technique was performed by our group and the study included 420 eyes in 370 patients (aged 25–60 years); 348 eyes with primary pterygium and 72 with recurrent pterygium. Results were excellent and recurrence rate was reported at 0.2%.[62]

4.8.4 Subconjunctival Excision of the Pterygium and MMC

This is one of our favorite techniques as it is minimally invasive, less time consuming, and is associated in our hands to an extremely low recurrence rate.[63] It consists in the dissection of the pterygium under the conjunctiva following the subconjunctival injection of saline and lidocaine 2% in the patient under local anesthesia. Then, the pterygium head is dissected by either tearing of the pterygium's head assisted by a crescent knife while the rest of the pterygium is dissected down to the insertion of the medial rectus muscle. Cautery hemostasis is made convenient, and then MMC

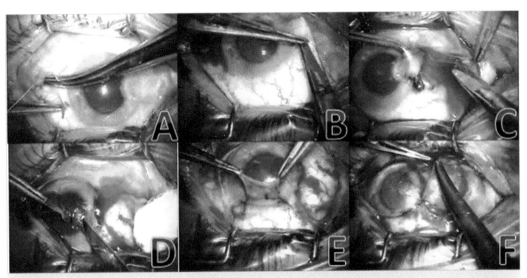

Fig. 4.1 Surgical steps of tailored corneo-conjunctival autografting: (**a**) traction suture, (**b**) dissection of the conjunctiva, (**c**) hooking the pterygium, (**d**) dissection of the pterygium from posterior to anterior and peeling the corneal part of the pterygium, (**e**) preparing the corneo-conjunctival graft, and (**f**) securing the graft with continuous nylon 10/0 suture.

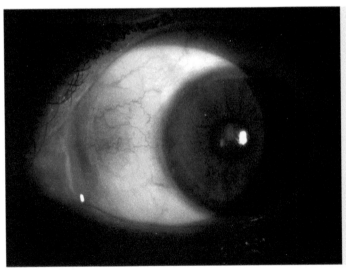

Fig. 4.2 A case of tailored corneo-conjunctival autografting 6 months postoperative.

0.02% is applied with a sponge placed subconjunctivally. Surgery is finished with 2 to 4 nylon 10/0 stitches replacing anatomically the conjunctival borders. Our results were published in 2008 and were associated to an extremely low recurrence rate.[63] This technique can also be used when dealing with reoperations. In such cases, we frequently use MMC at the same concentration preoperatively as a preparation for the reoperation surgery, as it

has been mentioned before in this chapter. Subconjunctival pterygium excision with intraoperative application of MMC seems to be, in our opinion, more anatomically driven allows better wound healing with less conjunctival scarring, and is associated with a very low reoperation rate due to its conservative anatomical and minimally invasive characteristics. Further long-term studies on this anatomical technique seem to be warranted.

References

[1] Detorakis ET, Spandidos DA. Pathogenetic mechanisms and treatment options for ophthalmic pterygium: trends and perspectives (Review). Int J Mol Med. 2009; 23(4): 439–447

[2] Hirst LW. The treatment of pterygium. Surv Ophthalmol. 2003; 48(2):145–180

[3] Martins TG, Costa AL, Alves MR, Chammas R, Schor P. Mitomycin C in pterygium treatment. Int J Ophthalmol. 2016; 9 (3):465–468

[4] Ozer A, Yildirim N, Erol N, Yurdakul S. Long-term results of bare sclera, limbal-conjunctival autograft and amniotic membrane graft techniques in primary pterygium excisions. Ophthalmologica. 2009; 223(4):269–273

[5] Jaros PA, DeLuise VP. Pingueculae and pterygia. Surv Ophthalmol. 1988; 33(1):41–49

[6] Singh G, Wilson MR, Foster CS. Long-term follow-up study of mitomycin eye drops as adjunctive treatment of pterygia and its comparison with conjunctival autograft transplantation. Cornea. 1990; 9(4):331–334

[7] D'Ombrain A. D'Ombrain A. The surgical treatment of pterygium. Br J Ophthalmol. 1948; 32(2):65–71

[8] Kenyon KR, Wagoner MD, Hettinger ME. Conjunctival autograft transplantation for advanced and recurrent pterygium. Ophthalmology. 1985; 92(11):1461–1470

[9] Janson BJ, Sikder S. Surgical management of pterygium. Ocul Surf. 2014; 12(2):112–119

[10] Nassiri N, Farahangiz S, Rahnavardi M, Rahmani L, Nassiri N. Corneal endothelial cell injury induced by mitomycin-C in photorefractive keratectomy: nonrandomized controlled trial. J Cataract Refract Surg. 2008; 34(6):902–908

[11] Avisar R, Avisar I, Bahar I, Weinberger D. Effect of mitomycin C in pterygium surgery on corneal endothelium. Cornea. 2008; 27(5):559–561

[12] Biswas MC, Shaw C, Mandal R, Islam MN, Chakroborty M. Treatment of pterygium with conjunctival limbal autograft and mitomycin C–a comparative study. J Indian Med Assoc. 2007; 105(4):200–, 202, 204

[13] Mutlu FM, Sobaci G, Tatar T, Yildirim E. A comparative study of recurrent pterygium surgery: limbal conjunctival autograft transplantation versus mitomycin C with conjunctival flap. Ophthalmology. 1999; 106(4):817–821

[14] Rodriguez JA, Ferrari C, Hernández GA. Intraoperative application of topical mitomycin C 0.05% for pterygium surgery. Bol Asoc Med P R. 2004; 96(2):100–102

[15] Tsai YY, Lin JM, Shy JD. Acute scleral thinning after pterygium excision with intraoperative mitomycin C: a case report of scleral dellen after bare sclera technique and review of the literature. Cornea. 2002; 21(2):227–229

[16] Young AL, Ho M, Jhanji V, Cheng LL. Ten-year results of a randomized controlled trial comparing 0.02% mitomycin C and limbal conjunctival autograft in pterygium surgery. Ophthalmology. 2013; 120(12):2390–2395

[17] Gupta VP, Saxena T. Comparison of single-drop mitomycin C regime with other mitomycin C regimes in pterygium surgery. Indian J Ophthalmol. 2003; 51(1):59–65

[18] Cheng HC, Tseng SH, Kao PL, Chen FK. Low-dose intraoperative mitomycin C as chemoadjuvant for pterygium surgery. Cornea. 2001; 20(1):24–29

[19] Raiskup F, Solomon A, Landau D, Ilsar M, Frucht-Pery J. Mitomycin C for pterygium: long term evaluation. Br J Ophthalmol. 2004; 88(11):1425–1428

[20] Chan TC, Wong RL, Li EY, et al. Twelve-year outcomes of pterygium excision with conjunctival autograft versus intra-operative mitomycin C in double-head pterygium Surgery. J Ophthalmol. 2015; 2015:891582

[21] Ma DH, See LC, Hwang YS, Wang SF. Comparison of amniotic membrane graft alone or combined with intraoperative mitomycin C to prevent recurrence after excision of recurrent pterygia. Cornea. 2005; 24(2):141–150

[22] Yanyali AC, Talu H, Alp BN, Karabas L, Ay GM, Caglar Y. Intra-operative mitomycin C in the treatment of pterygium. Cornea. 2000; 19(4):471–473

[23] Mohammed I. Treatment of pterygium. Ann Afr Med. 2011; 10(3):197–203

[24] Kheirkhah A, Hashemi H, Adelpour M, Nikdel M, Rajabi MB, Behrouz MJ. Randomized trial of pterygium surgery with mitomycin C application using conjunctival autograft versus conjunctival-limbal autograft. Ophthalmology. 2012; 119(2): 227–232

[25] Sharma A, Gupta A, Ram J, Gupta A. Low-dose intraoperative mitomycin-C versus conjunctival autograft in primary pterygium surgery: long term follow-up. Ophthalmic Surg Lasers. 2000; 31(4):301–307

[26] Ang LP, Chua JL, Tan DT. Current concepts and techniques in pterygium treatment. Curr Opin Ophthalmol. 2007; 18(4): 308–313

[27] Hosal BM, Gursel E. Mitomycin-C for prevention of recurrent pterygium. Ann Ophthalmol- Glaucoma. 2000; 32:107–109

[28] Oguz H, Basar E, Gurler B. Intraoperative application versus postoperative mitomycin C eye drops in pterygium surgery. Acta Ophthalmol Scand. 1999; 77(2):147–150

[29] Frucht-Pery J, Raiskup F, Ilsar M, Landau D, Orucov F, Solomon A. Conjunctival autografting combined with low-dose mitomycin C for prevention of primary pterygium recurrence. Am J Ophthalmol. 2006; 141(6):1044–1050

[30] Keklikci U, Celik Y, Cakmak SS, Unlu MK, Bilek B. Conjunctival-limbal autograft, amniotic membrane transplantation, and intraoperative mitomycin C for primary pterygium. Ann Ophthalmol (Skokie). 2007; 39(4):296–301

[31] Rahman A, Yahya K, Ul Hasan KS. Recurrence rate of pterygium following surgical excision with intraoperative versus postoperative mitomycin-C. J Coll Physicians Surg Pak. 2008; 18(8):489–492

[32] Ari S, Caca I, Yildiz ZO, Sakalar YB, Dogan E. Comparison of mitomycin C and limbal-conjunctival autograft in the prevention of pterygial recurrence in Turkish patients: a one-year, randomized, assessor-masked, controlled trial. Curr Ther Res Clin Exp. 2009; 70(4):274–281

[33] Mahar PS, Manzar N. Pterygium recurrence related to its size and corneal involvement. J Coll Physicians Surg Pak. 2013; 23 (2):120–123

[34] Thakur SK, Khaini KR, Panda A. Role of low dose mitomycin C in pterygium surgery. Nepal J Ophthalmol. 2012; 4(1):203–205

[35] Narsani AK, Jatoi SM, Gul S, Dabir SA. Treatment of primary pterygium with conjunctival autograft and mitomycin C A comparative study. J Liaquat Uni Med Health Sci. 2008; 7(4): 184–187

[36] Avisar R, Apel I, Avisar I, Weinberger D. Endothelial cell loss during pterygium surgery: importance of timing of mitomycin C application. Cornea. 2009; 28(8):879–881

[37] Young AL, Tam PM, Leung GY, Cheng LL, Lam PT, Lam DS. Prospective study on the safety and efficacy of combined conjunctival rotational autograft with intraoperative 0.02% mitomycin C in primary pterygium excision. Cornea. 2009; 28(2):166–169

[38] Koranyi G, Artzén D, Seregard S, Kopp ED. Intraoperative mitomycin C versus autologous conjunctival autograft in

surgery of primary pterygium with four-year follow-up. Acta Ophthalmol. 2012; 90(3):266–270

[39] Zaky KS, Khalifa YM. Efficacy of preoperative injection versus intraoperative application of mitomycin in recurrent pterygium surgery. Indian J Ophthalmol. 2012; 60(4):273–276

[40] Donnenfeld ED, Perry HD, Fromer S, Doshi S, Solomon R, Biser S. Subconjunctival mitomycin C as adjunctive therapy before pterygium excision. Ophthalmology. 2003; 110(5):1012–1016

[41] Levy J, Tessler Z, Rosenthal G, et al. Toxic effects of subconjunctival 5-fluorouracil and mitomycin C on ciliary body of rats. Int Ophthalmol. 2001; 24(4):199–203

[42] Strong B, Farley W, Stern ME, Pflugfelder SC. Topical cyclosporine inhibits conjunctival epithelial apoptosis in experimental murine keratoconjunctivitis sicca. Cornea. 2005; 24(1):80–85

[43] Ibáñez M, Eugarrios MF, Calderón DI. Topical cyclosporin A and mitomycin C injection as adjunctive therapy for prevention of primary pterygium recurrence. Ophthalmic Surg Lasers Imaging. 2009; 40(3):239–244

[44] Turan-Vural E, Torun-Acar B, Kivanc SA, Acar S. The effect of topical 0.05% cyclosporine on recurrence following pterygium surgery. Clin Ophthalmol. 2011; 5:881–885

[45] Yalcin Tok O, Burcu Nurozler A, Ergun G, Akbas Kocaoglu F, Duman S. Topical cyclosporine A in the prevention of pterygium recurrence. Ophthalmologica. 2008; 222(6):391–396

[46] Ozgurhan EB, Agca A, Kara N, Yuksel K, Demircan A, Demirok A. Topical application of bevacizumab as an adjunct to recurrent pterygium surgery. Cornea. 2013; 32(6):835–838

[47] Lazic R, Gabric N. Intravitreally administered bevacizumab (Avastin) in minimally classic and occult choroidal neovascularization secondary to age-related macular degeneration. Graefes Arch Clin Exp Ophthalmol. 2007; 245(1):68–73

[48] Jorge R, Costa RA, Calucci D, Cintra LP, Scott IU. Intravitreal bevacizumab (Avastin) for persistent new vessels in diabetic retinopathy (IBEPE study). Retina. 2006; 26(9):1006–1013

[49] Stevenson W, Cheng SF, Dastjerdi MH, Ferrari G, Dana R. Corneal neovascularization and the utility of topical VEGF inhibition: ranibizumab (Lucentis) vs bevacizumab (Avastin). Ocul Surf. 2012; 10(2):67–83

[50] Chen JJ, Ebmeier SE, Sutherland WM, Ghazi NG. Potential penetration of topical ranibizumab (Lucentis) in the rabbit eye. Eye (Lond). 2011; 25(11):1504–1511

[51] Motarjemizadeh Q, Aidenloo NS, Sepehri S. A comparative study of different concentrations of topical bevacizumab on the recurrence rate of excised primary pterygium: a short-term follow-up study. Int Ophthalmol. 2016; 36(1):63–71

[52] Suh JS, Choi SK. The effect of subconjunctival bevacizumab injection after primary pterygium surgery. J Korean Ophthalmol Soc. 2013; 54:53–59

[53] Ali AM, Thariat J, Bensadoun RJ, et al. The role of radiotherapy in the treatment of pterygium: a review of the literature including more than 6000 treated lesions. Cancer Radiother. 2011; 15(2):140–147

[54] Koch JM, Mellin KB, Waubke TN. [The pterygium, autologous conjunctiva-limbus transplantation as treatment]. Ophthalmologe. 1992; 89(2):143–146

[55] Figueiredo RS, Cohen EJ, Gomes JAP, Rapuano CJ, Laibson PR. Conjunctival autograft for pterygium surgery: how well does it prevent recurrence? Ophthalmic Surg Lasers. 1997; 28(2):99–104

[56] Xi XH, Jiang DY, Tang LS. [Transplantation of amniotic membrane and amniotic membrane combined with limbal autograft for patients with complicated pterygium]. Hunan Yi Ke Da Xue Xue Bao. 2003; 28(2):149–151

[57] Dua HS, Azuara-Blanco A. Amniotic membrane transplantation. Br J Ophthalmol. 1999; 83(6):748–752

[58] Meller D, Pauklin M, Thomasen H, Westekemper H, Steuhl K-P. Amniotic membrane transplantation in the human eye. Dtsch Arztebl Int. 2011; 108(14):243–248

[59] Rahman I, Said DG, Maharajan VS, Dua HS. Amniotic membrane in ophthalmology: indications and limitations. Eye (Lond). 2009; 23(10):1954–1961

[60] Chui J, Di Girolamo N, Wakefield D, Coroneo MT. The pathogenesis of pterygium: current concepts and their therapeutic implications. Ocul Surf. 2008; 6(1):24–43

[61] Hernández-Bogantes E, Amescua G, Navas A, et al. Minor ipsilateral simple limbal epithelial transplantation (mini-SLET) for pterygium treatment. Br J Ophthalmol. 2015; 99(12):1598–1600

[62] Genidy MM, Abdelghany AA, Alio JL. Tailored corneo-conjunctival autografting in primary and secondary pterygium surgery. Eur J Ophthalmol. 2017; 27(4):407–410

[63] de la Hoz F, Montero JA, Alió JL, Javaloy J, Ruiz-Moreno JM, Sala E. Efficacy of mitomycin C associated with direct conjunctival closure and sliding conjunctival graft for pterygium surgery. Br J Ophthalmol. 2008; 92(2):175–178

5 Ocular Surface and Tear Film Management in Pterygium Surgery

Alanna S. Nattis, Henry D. Perry, and Eric D. Donnenfeld

Abstract

The evolution of pterygium surgery continues as we learn more about the interaction of ocular surface inflammation, dry eye, and factors influencing clinical, anatomical, and surgical success. Good surgical technique is the foundation for success; however, management of dry eye, meibomian gland dysfunction (MGD), and blepharitis should not be ignored.[1] Inflammation associated with ocular surface disease may create a feedback mechanism via release of cytokines and growth factors that stimulate pterygium growth and recurrence. Herein, we review the impact of poor ocular surface health and inflammation, in its relation to pterygium surgery.

Keywords: pterygium, dry eye, meibomian gland dysfunction, ocular surface disease, cytokines, growth factors, recurrence

5.1 Introduction

A pterygium is usually a triangular encroachment of the nasal bulbar conjunctiva onto the cornea and is derived from the Greek word for "little wing."[1,2,3] It is a degenerative and hyperplastic process with invasion of the peripheral cornea to the level of Bowman's membrane.[1] Pterygium is a worldwide external disease problem and is especially common in the "pterygium belt," 10 to 30 degrees above and below the equator.[1,2] This geographic area is characterized by greater exposure to sunlight and ultraviolet (UV) radiation, as well as to dry, dusty, and strong winds, which are thought to be integral to pterygium pathogenesis.[1,2,3,4] Although more common in men, in areas with equal sun exposure (e.g., Aruba), the incidence for men and women is similar.[1] In the northern climes, pterygium is much less common and mostly limited to patients with vocations that are exclusive to outdoor work.[1,2] Dry eye disease and ocular surface inflammation are thought to be adjunctive factors.[1,5,6] There is no well-defined inheritance pattern, but the tendency toward pterygia appears to be autosomal dominant with low penetrance.[1,7] The growth of the pterygia is toward the center of the cornea and can, though rarely, cross the visual axis.[1,2,6,8] Extensive growth of a pterygium up to and partially through the visual axis is shown in ▶ Fig. 5.1.

The tendency for the nasal conjunctiva being involved in the vast majority of cases is thought to be secondary to increased UV damage (possibly from reflection off the nose or the passage of light through the anterior chamber).[1,9] When temporal and nasal pterygia coexist in one eye ("double headed"), the temporal pterygium usually forms later.[1,2,6,8] An example of a double-headed pterygium is shown in ▶ Fig. 5.2.

A conservative, non-surgical approach may be taken with small pterygia that do not involve much of the cornea.[2] However, for larger pterygia causing visual disturbances, restriction of eye

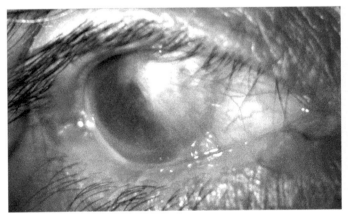

Fig. 5.1 Extensive pterygium crossing through the visual axis.

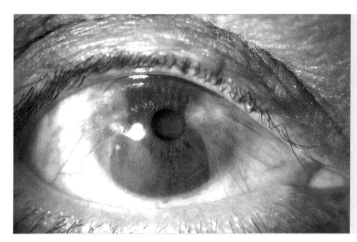

Fig. 5.2 "Double-headed" (nasal and temporal) pterygium.

movement, unacceptable cosmesis, occurrence of secondary degenerative changes, or persistent irritation, the standard of care regarding pterygium management is surgical excision.[1,2,5] Different techniques have been developed in the realm of pterygium surgery, all with different indications, risks, and recurrence rates.[1,2,3,4,5,6,8,9,10,11,12,13,14,15,16,17] Of interest are factors that lead to, and that importantly, can prevent pterygium recurrence, saving the patient additional surgery as well as cost to the healthcare system.[1,2,3,5,6,8,9,10,11,12,13,14,15,18,19,20,21,22,23,24,25,26]

There is extensive literature citing increased levels of ocular surface inflammation in the formation, growth, and recurrence of pterygia.[5,6,20,21,27,28,29,30] Several inflammatory markers found in dry eye disease are also found in eyes with primary and recurrent pterygia.[5,6,27,28,29,30] Thus, it is important to understand the pathogenesis of dry eye and ocular surface disease as it relates to the formation of pterygia, in order to properly manage these patients postoperatively, improve comfort, and prevent recurrences. Too often, common sense approaches, such as wearing a hat or polarized lenses outdoors, are ignored.

5.2 Pterygium Anatomy and Histology

There are three distinct parts of the pterygium. The cap or leading edge consists of a flat gray zone on the cornea, consisting mainly of fibroblasts—this area invades and destroys Bowman's membrane.[1,31] An iron line (*Stocker's line*) may be seen anterior to the cap; there may be a dellen anterior

to the cap.[1] The pterygium head is immediately behind the cap and consists of a whitish, thickened vascular area firmly attached to the cornea.[1,31] The body ("tail") is a fleshy, mobile vascular area of bulbar conjunctiva and serves as an important landmark for surgical dissection.[1] Tan et al developed an anatomically based grading system for pterygia, which was predictive of recurrence.[2,32] The three types they identified were T1 (atrophic; episcleral vessels underlying pterygium are unobscured), T2 (intermediate; episcleral vessels are partially obscured), and T3 (fleshy; thick pterygium in which episcleral vessels underlying the body of the pterygium are totally obscured by fibrovascular tissue), T3 being the variant with the highest recurrence risk.[2,32] Examples of the clinical types of pterygia are shown in ▶ Fig. 5.3, ▶ Fig. 5.4, ▶ Fig. 5.5.

The histopathology of pterygia has been compared to that of pinguecula inasmuch as both lesions are characterized by elastotic degeneration of the stroma.[1,31] However, when compared to pterygia, pinguecula tend to be relatively poorly vascularized.[1,31] Both lesions originate from activated fibroblasts thought to occur from actinic stimulation and are more common on the nasal surface of the limbal conjunctiva in the interpalpebral area.[1,2] On histologic evaluation, the stroma shows increased fibroblasts, pockets of inflammatory cells, and prominent hyalinization of stromal fibrils with increased amounts of twisted fibers that stain positively for elastic tissue, but resist digestion with elastase, hence the term *elastotic degeneration*.[1,31] In some areas, there may be eosinophilic and basophilic changes that can simulate concretions.[1,2,31] The epithelium can transform

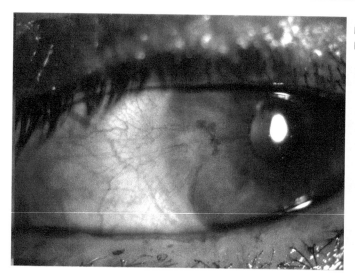

Fig. 5.3 Atrophic (T1), thin, small pterygium.

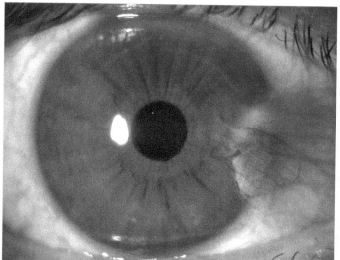

Fig. 5.4 Intermediate (T2) pterygium.

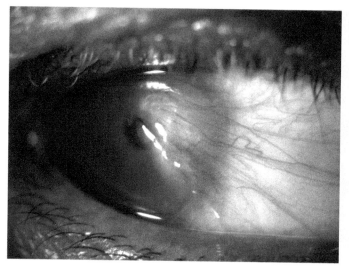

Fig. 5.5 Large, thickened (T3) pterygium.

into an acanthotic pattern that may have mild dysplastic areas and eventually in rare cases can lead to squamous cell carcinoma.[1,2,33,34] Other areas in the epithelium may present with hyperkeratosis or goblet cell proliferation.[1,2] The head of the pterygia has a fibrovascular frond that invades Bowman's membrane. The pterygium body has mostly basophilic areas that represent damaged fibroblasts and altered stromal fibrils (i.e., *elastotic degeneration*).[1,31]

5.3 Etiologies and Growth of Pterygia

The prevalence of pterygia has been reported to range from 0.3 to 29%.[9] Many theories are suggested in the etiology and pathogenesis of pterygia (UV light exposure and chronic irritation from dust/wind).[9] They may present as a visual disturbance due to induction of astigmatism or by its growth extending onto the cornea to occlude the visual axis.[9] It may cause ocular irritation/recurrent inflammation and be cosmetically unsightly.[9]

Pterygia typically grow in two stages: (1) the initial and progressive disruption of limbal corneal-conjunctival epithelial barrier and (2) progressive active "conjunctivalization" of the cornea by tissue characterized by extensive cellular proliferation, connective tissue remodeling, inflammation, and angiogenesis.[6] These factors can be managed individually and, if done successfully, can lead to excellent clinical and surgical outcomes in patients with pterygia.

As pterygia are thought to result from actinic damage and form from submucosal growth of fibrovascular connective tissue that migrates onto the cornea, they are viewed by some as aggressive growths with concern for dysplastic degeneration.[31] Additionally, impression cytology of surface cells directly overlying a pterygium has been shown to be abnormal, with increased goblet cell density and squamous metaplasia.[1,21,31]

Fortunately, most pterygia are entirely benign; it is worthwhile sending the excised tissue for pathologic examination, because occasionally, precursors of actinic-induced neoplasms (e.g., squamous cell carcinoma and melanoma) are detected.[1,31]

5.4 Surgical Management

The main consideration with pterygia is regarding treatment, when to operate and how to best manage patients postoperatively. Historically, the initial treatment has been simple removal ("bare sclera technique"). Unfortunately, this has been associated with a recurrence rate of 40 to 90%.[7] This unacceptable recurrence rate has led to dozens of surgical techniques and the use of adjunctive agents such as mitomycin C (MMC), 5-fluorouracil (5-FU), and others.[2] Through the research of Friend and Thoft, the concept of conjunctival transplantation was born.[1,2,35,36] This change in therapy led to an increase in success rate, decreased recurrences and obviates for the most part, and the use of dangerous adjunctive alkylating agents.[1,2,35,36]

Some of the therapies that have been popular include bare sclera technique with and without beta-radiation, pterygium excision with a mobile flap, mucous membrane graft, skin graft, misdirection of the head of the pterygium, lamellar scleral grafts, amniotic membrane, limbal conjunctival autografts, and free conjunctival autografts.[1,2] Many surgeons have incorporated the use of tissue transplantation (i.e., amniotic membrane and conjunctival grafts) after pterygium excision in an effort to reduce recurrence. These grafts may be sutured in place or glued (e.g., fibrin glue and autologous blood).[10]

5.5 Surgical Techniques

Herein, we briefly describe past and current techniques for pterygium excision. From bare sclera to the pterygium-extended removal followed by extended conjunctival transplant (PERFECT) technique, the techniques listed below are in order of increasing success rate and decreasing recurrence rate, as defined by the literature.[2,4,5,8,9,11,12,13,14,16,26,37,38]

5.5.1 Bare Sclera

D'ombrian introduced the Bare Sclera technique in 1948; this technique is generally considered inadequate secondary to high recurrence rates.[2] Pterygium is excised in toto, and the sclera is left bare without graft or primary closure.

5.5.2 Lamellar Keratectomy

Lamellar keratectomy is mainly reserved for recurrent pterygia with scarred or thin corneal tissue.[9] After surgery for recurrent pterygium, there may be significant residual scarring and thinning of the cornea.[13] In this case, lamellar corneal graft tissue can be used to replace thin or scarred portions of the cornea.[13]

5.5.3 Primary Conjunctival Closure and Sliding/Rotational Conjunctival Flaps

Primary conjunctival closure and sliding/rotational conjunctival flaps has also been used, but recurrence rates do not appear to be significantly better than the bare sclera technique (29–37%).[2,5,9] Here, either sliding conjunctival flaps from both the superior and inferior limbus, or a rotation of a flap of superior conjunctiva is sutured or glued into place.[2,5,9]

5.5.4 Amniotic membrane grafts

Amniotic membrane grafts have been shown to be more efficacious than bare sclera technique, but have higher recurrence rates than conjunctival autografts (approximately 14–28%).[5,8,11] However, amniotic membrane may be preferable in patients who do not have adequate tissue available for transplantation (e.g., multiple prior surgeries with conjunctival scarring, those with filtering blebs, or those who may need glaucoma filtration surgery in the future).[5] Amniotic membrane is thought to promote healing and to reduce rates of recurrence through its anti-inflammatory properties.[8] Amniotic membrane may help suppress transforming growth factor-beta (TGF-β), and thus act as an antifibrotic agent.[5] It also acts as a basement membrane substance that allows epithelium to grow over it, perhaps speeding the healing process.[3,6] We have seen its successful use in severe ocular surface disease, ocular burns, and forniceal reconstruction in limbal stem cell deficiency.[8] As some feel that the etiology of pterygium is related to localized limbal stem cell deficiency, and that this condition may be exacerbated by dry eye, amniotic membrane is a logical choice for use during pterygium excision.[8] Additionally, amniotic membrane has been shown to inhibit inflammation by releasing anti-inflammatory cytokines from its epithelium and stroma (interleukin [IL]-10 and IL-1 receptor antagonists).[8] In concert with these findings, amniotic membrane has been shown to decrease postoperative pain and rarely has problems with tissue rejection, as it does not express human leukocyte antigen (HLA) surface proteins (i.e., HLA-A, HLA-B, and HLA-D-rerated [HLA-DR]).[6]

5.5.5 Conjunctival Limbal Autograft

Conjunctival limbal autograft is a useful technique in pterygium surgery, as one of the proposed etiologies of pterygium is focal limbal stem cell deficiency.[2] The procedure is similar to that of obtaining a conjunctival autograft; however, the limbal edge of the donor graft is extended to include limbal epithelium, either by superficial keratectomy or superficial lamellar dissection.[2,3,6] The graft is then secured in place with glue or sutures.

5.5.6 Free Conjunctival Autografts

Free conjunctival autografts provide the lowest rate of recurrence and have even been shown to be successful when split in half for use with double-headed pterygia.[5,13] Typically, the free graft is obtained from the superotemporal conjunctiva and is placed over the bare scleral bed following pterygium excision.[2] Many studies have shown this technique to be superior to amniotic membrane transplantation, among others.[2,5,6,8,9,11,12,14,26] Conjunctival autografting is widely used as a tissue replacement after pterygium excision as it is readily available and has been shown to have excellent anatomical and functional results.[2,5] The autograft provides a source of healthy conjunctival epithelium and may act by *contact inhibition* on the residual abnormal tissue to prevent recurrence.[5,26] In addition, placing the conjunctival autograft in a limbus-to-limbus orientation may yield a better result by acting as a barrier against fibrovascular invasion of the cornea and supplying stem cells to the corneal epithelium.[2,5] Bare sclera at the site of pterygium excision has been suggested to serve as a scaffold for pterygium regrowth and recurrence, either by induction of a dellen, or by expression of inflammatory cytokines.[5]

5.5.7 Pterygium-Extended Removal Followed by Extended Conjunctival Transplant

PERFECT, developed by Hirst, is a very successful, although extensive procedure for pterygium excision.[2,4,16,37] In this technique, there is wide excision of Tenon's capsule above and below and over the corresponding rectus muscle (e.g., medial rectus for nasal pterygium and lateral rectus for temporal pterygium).[2,4,16,37] For a nasal pterygium, there is subsequent excision of the semilunar fold, which leaves a very large defect.[2,4,16] The defect is then covered by an extensive, thin, free conjunctival graft.[2,4,16,37] This technique has been shown to be extremely successful with close to zero recurrence rates, even in double-headed pterygia.[2,4,16,37]

5.6 Adjunctive Therapies for Pterygium Excision

In high-risk cases (increased risk of recurrence or surgery for recurrent pterygium), adjunctive therapy may be used to help prevent recurrence.[2,5,8,11] These therapies include use of alkylating agents (MMC and 5-FU), anti-vascular endothelial growth factor (anti-VEGF), alcohol, and others.[2,8,9,14] Adjunctive therapy may be employed preoperatively, intraoperative, or postoperatively to enhance pterygium surgery success.[2,8,9,13,36] Unfortunately, the majority of these therapies may lead to late serious ocular sequelae.[2,3,9,10,17,36]

5.6.1 Beta-Irradiation

Beta-irradiation (Strontium-90) has reportedly reduced recurrence rates, via reducing the rate of proliferating cells in the wound bed.[3] However, there are a plethora of possible late complications, such as scleral melts, infectious scleritis, endophthalmitis, corneal perforation, cataract, iris atrophy, secondary glaucoma, calcific scleral plaque, conjunctivitis, keratitis, ptosis, and limbal stem cell deficiency (and resultant severe ocular surface disease).[2,9] This treatment has largely fallen out of favor in the United States, but is still in use in other countries.

5.6.2 Thiotepa

Thiotepa is a nitrogen mustard-alkylating agent with antimitotic properties that is thought to be able to obliterate proliferating vascular endothelial cells.[3] It was originally used in Japan in conjunction with the bare sclera technique, decreasing recurrence rates to approximately 12 to 16%.[3] However, this compound is also associated with adverse effects, such as prolonged conjunctival hyperemia, irritation, allergy, bacterial corneoscleritis, and permanent eyelid depigmentation.[3]

5.6.3 Corticosteroids

Corticosteroids, either given as a drop or via subconjunctival injection, have been found to be a useful adjunct in some cases in preventing recurrence.[8] Use of corticosteroids is thought to inhibit the inflammatory reaction induced by pterygium surgery and therefore reduces neovascularization at the operative site.[3] The dosing frequency and duration of treatment varies; corticosteroids may be used both preoperatively and/or postoperatively.[3]

5.6.4 Mitomycin C

MMC is an antibiotic derived from the bacteria *Streptomyces caespitosus*, and acts as an alkylating agent that inhibits cell division by inhibiting DNA, cellular RNA, and protein synthesis.[2,8,17] It is most commonly used intraoperatively, applied to bare sclera, but has also been used pre- and postoperatively.[2,8,9,17] MMC has a strong antiproliferative effect, owing to action on both fibroblasts and VEGF.[18] Research has shown that its adjunctive use has led to decreased recurrence rates with bare sclera, amniotic membrane graft, and conjunctival autograft techniques.[8,17]

5.6.5 5-Fluorouracil

5-FU is a pyrimidine analog that interferes with DNA and RNA synthesis.[2] It induces apoptosis of Tenon's fibroblasts, has anti-fibroblast activity, and may be used intraoperatively.[2,9] This medication is relatively affordable and is readily available compared to some other adjunctive therapies (e.g., anti-VEGF).[9] Although efficacious, it should be remembered that side effects of chemotherapeutic agents (e.g., MMC and 5-FU) are potentially serious and mimic those seen with beta-irradiation, including punctate epitheliopathy, increased intraocular pressure, and delayed onset scleral melt.[2,8,9]

5.6.6 Alcohol

Alcohol has been used as an adjunctive therapy, secondary to its ability to denature cytokines and growth factors, which may be involved in pterygium formation.[9] In addition, there have been studies demonstrating a decreased rate of recurrence and fewer postoperative complications comparing alcohol versus MMC as adjunctive therapy.[9]

5.6.7 Anti-VEGF

Anti-VEGF therapy has been employed as adjunctive treatment for pterygia and pterygia recurrence.[9] This therapy is of interest as pterygia exhibit significantly higher levels of VEGF than normal cornea and conjunctiva.[13] Thus, blocking VEGF may halt the vascularity and growth of pterygia.[13] In addition, anti-VEGF also reduces inflammation and thus may reduce pterygium symptoms (e.g., redness and irritation).[14] Bevacizumab (Avastin, Genentech Inc., San Francisco, CA) is an anti-VEGF recombinant humanized murine monoclonal IgG1 that inhibits the VEGF-A isoform, the predominant stimulant of angiogenesis.[13] Recently, a randomized clinical trial reported the use of subconjunctival bevacizumab in conjunction with primary pterygium excision with conjunctival autograft to be safe and well tolerated, as well as capable of preventing recurrence when compared to control.[9,13] There may also be a dose-dependence inhibitory effect of bevacizumab on cultured Tenon's fibroblasts, as studies have shown positive results with increased frequency of dosing, either via subconjunctival injection or topical eye drop administration.[13]

5.7 Role of Ocular Surface Health

In addition to induced astigmatism, potential limitation of extraocular motility, and binocular diplopia, pterygia can also impair vision through ·an altered tear film and epiphora.[6] The combination of pterygium and dry eye (either in coexistence or one exacerbating the other) can perpetuate the symptomatology and growth of pterygium, as well as its recurrence after surgery.[6,15,18] This fact leads us to perform a detailed dry eye evaluation in all our pterygia patients. It becomes obvious that maintenance of a healthy ocular surface and tear film is essential in these patients for optimal anatomical, clinical, and surgical outcomes.

In a study by Kampitak et al, it was determined that eyes that were post-pterygium excision with amniotic membrane who received lubrication therapy with artificial tears had a significantly lower recurrence rate (16%) compared to the control group (33%).[18] Additionally, double-headed pterygia have been found to be associated with dry eye.[15] These findings and others lead us to aggressively treat our patients for their associated dry eye disease.

Multiple studies have examined different dry eye symptoms and parameters (tear osmolarity [TOT]), tear breakup time (TBUT), Schirmer's testing, corneal staining, and their relation to pterygium growth, symptomatology, and recurrence.[19,20,21,22,23,24,25,29,30] Schirmer's and TBUT scores in pterygium patients are significantly reduced compared to those in controls, suggesting that both aqueous and mucin deficiency of the ocular surface may be inciting factors for pterygium growth.[19,20,21,29,30] In addition, improvement in TBUT, tear ferning tests and goblet cell densities have been shown post pterygium excision, demonstrating that tear function in patients with pterygium has a close relationship to dry eye, and that the presence of pterygium may initiate or exacerbate its symptoms.[21,25] In most cases, there is evidence of surface irritation on examination, as seen in ▶ Fig. 5.6, ▶ Fig. 5.7, ▶ Fig. 5.8.

TOT has also been shown to improve post pterygium excision and deteriorate with pterygium recurrence.[27,39] Thus, it is not only imperative to provide good surgical outcomes in these patients, but also to optimize the ocular surface of these patients in order to prevent recurrence.[21] It becomes clear that maintenance of a stable ocular surface in pterygium patients can help prevent further growth and possibly prevent the need for surgery in some cases.

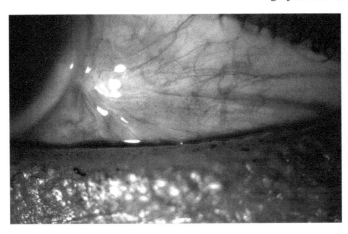

Fig. 5.6 Lissamine green staining on the surface of a pterygium.

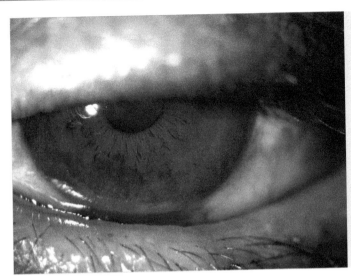

Fig. 5.7 Severe dry eye enhanced by Lissamine green stain.

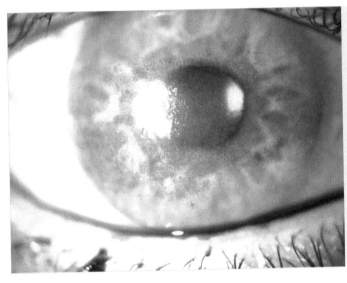

Fig. 5.8 Severe dry eye with intense corneal staining.

Studies of the eyelids and meibomian gland health regarding pterygium growth and recurrence have shown that poor eyelid health is correlated with worsening pterygium symptoms and recurrences.[28] Meibomian gland function has been recognized as a critical factor in maintaining the health and stability of the ocular surface.[28,40] Meibomian glands make and secrete lipid, which distributes across the ocular surface, becoming the outermost layer of the tear film.[28,40] With meibomian gland dysfunction (MGD), there is terminal blockage of the glands, and/or abnormalities of materials/secretion quality, leading to evaporative dry eye.[28,40] Examples of MGD are shown in ▶ Fig. 5.9 and ▶ Fig. 5.10.

Decreased meibomian gland function has been correlated with progressive pterygium versus those with stable MGD and stable pterygium.[28] The combination of altered tear dynamics and chronic ocular surface inflammation appear to promote pterygium growth.[28] Additionally, the presence of pterygium, MGD, and tear film abnormalities appear to feed upon each other, causing a cycle of irritation and inflammation on an already irregular ocular surface, also promoting pterygium growth.[28] Thus, while treating dry eye and ocular surface disease in pterygium patients, either pre- or postoperatively, it is important to develop a treatment plan for adequate surface lubrication and maintenance of meibomian gland function and eyelid hygiene.

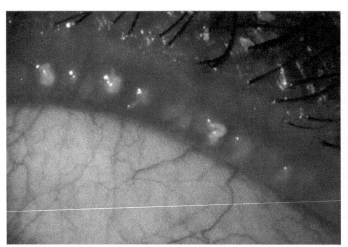

Fig. 5.9 Meibomian gland dysfunction (MGD): irregular gland expression/product.

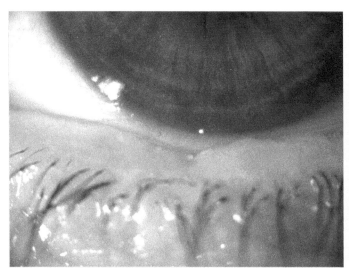

Fig. 5.10 Advanced meibomian gland dysfunction (MGD) with lid notching and irregular contour of lid margin.

Another factor that has been linked to pterygium formation and recurrence is the presence of demodicosis (infestation of Demodex folliculorum [lashes] and Demodex brevis [within meibomian glands]).[27] These parasites are associated with recalcitrant blepharitis and MGD, producing, in some cases significant ocular surface disease, irritation, and dry eye.[27] Often, patients with demodicosis demonstrate a classic "cylindrical dandruff" present at the eyelash base, significant lid crusting, and matting of the eyelashes. Examples of this are shown in ▶ Fig. 5.11 and ▶ Fig. 5.12.

In a report by Huang et al, 94 patients with pterygia and confirmed demodicosis were evaluated for recurrence rate and IL-17 levels.[27] IL-17 (mainly secreted by CD4 T-cells [Th17 lympho-cytes]) is a key cytokine involved in chronic inflammatory disease with and without autoimmune dysregulation.[27] Tear levels of IL-17 have been noted to be elevated in several chronic inflammatory conditions, such as filamentary keratitis, graft versus host disease, autoimmune keratitis, Sjögren's syndrome, dry eye, MGD, and Stevens–Johnson syndrome.[27] It was found that ocular demodicosis was more prevalent in patients with recurrent pterygium versus primary pterygium; these patients also had a significantly higher level of IL-17 compared with controls.[27] The authors concluded that ocular demodicosis was a risk factor for pterygium recurrence, further highlighting the importance of maintenance of the ocular surface and eyelid hygiene for pterygium prevention and care.[27]

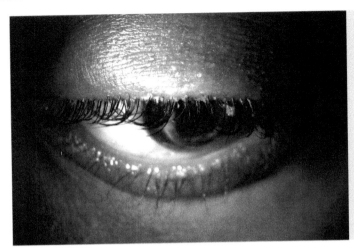

Fig. 5.11 Blepharitis and lash crusting associated with demodicosis.

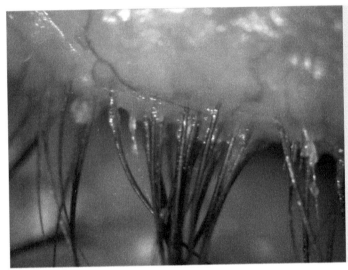

Fig. 5.12 Cylindrical dandruff and lash crusting in a patient with demodicosis.

Corneal limbal stem cells are usually abnormal in pterygia, such that the limbal corneal conjunctival epithelial barrier is disrupted, and the cornea assumes conjunctival characteristics in a process marked by extensive cellular proliferation, inflammation, connective tissue remodeling, and angiogenesis.[6] Intact corneal epithelium plays an essential role in corneal clarity and function.[6,27] It is continuously renewed by a population of epithelial limbal stem cells that are located at the basal limbus.[6,27] A healthy limbus acts as a barrier to conjunctival overgrowth, thus inclusion of healthy tissue from grafting may reduce pterygium recurrence both physically and physiologically.[6] Classic signs and symptoms of limbal stem cell deficiency include conjunctival ingrowth, vascularization, chronic inflammation, destruction of basement membrane, and fibrous ingrowth—all are clearly present in pterygia, leading researchers to suggest that pterygium is a manifestation of localized interpalpebral limbal stem cell deficiency, perhaps as a consequence of UV light–related stem cell destruction.[2,41] An example of limbal stem cell deficiency is seen in ▶ Fig. 5.13.

In concert with this, studies have shown that healing of the ocular surface is expedited with adequate lubrication and that severely dry eyes often have deficient healing properties, as is seen in limbal stem cell deficiency.[6] Highlighting the importance of limbal stem cells, conjunctival autografts that contain limbal stem cells have been shown to reduce recurrence rates in pterygium patients compared with amniotic membrane transplantation.[6]

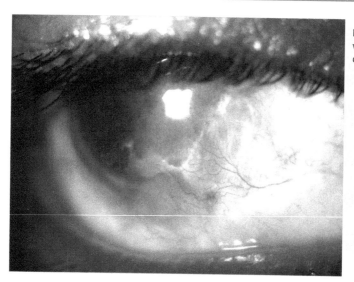

Fig. 5.13 Limbal stem cell deficiency with corneal neovascularization and conjunctivalization.

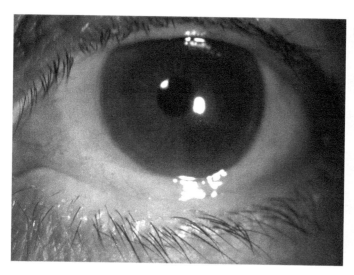

Fig. 5.14 Conjunctivochalasis.

Abnormal structural properties of the ocular surface may also play a role in pterygium formation. Tong et al suggest that conjunctivochalasis, a condition whose prevalence increases with age and is associated with redundancy of the conjunctival epithelium and stroma, may be a precursor to pterygia.[42] Upon inspection of a patient with conjunctivochalasis, one can clinically observe excess and parallel folds of conjunctiva that can disrupt tear flow and even encroach on the cornea.[42] Examples of conjunctivochalasis are shown in ▶ Fig. 5.14 and ▶ Fig. 5.15.

Both pterygium and conjunctivochalasis are associated with inflammatory changes and elastic tissue abnormalities that promote inflammatory matrix metalloproteinases (MMPs), which may be key to the invasive behavior of the pterygium head.[42] The theory behind this idea is that if loose conjunctiva is allowed to overhang the cornea, but not adhere, as in some forms of conjunctivochalasis, and there are additional factors causing irritation and inflammation of the ocular surface (UV irradiation, recurrent trauma, and dry eye), the conjunctival epithelial cells may produce MMPs and cause localized breakdown of corneal epithelium down to Bowman's membrane.[42] This would allow the newly formed pterygium head to fuse to the cornea and form the highly adherent pterygium apex.[42] This theory also suggests that treatment of conjunctivochalasis before it possibly transforms into pterygium (e.g., anti-inflammatory measures, avoidance of UV light) may be

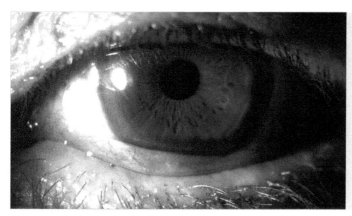

Fig. 5.15 Conjunctivochalasis and resultant ocular surface irritation/dry eye as highlighted by Lissamine green stain.

beneficial.[42] Lastly, during pterygium resection, it may not be necessary to perform too extensive of a resection, as this can remove relatively normal conjunctiva.[42]

5.7.1 Role of Inflammation

It is known that pterygia are associated with inflammation, as are ocular surface disease and dry eye. Together, these entities may perpetuate each other, and thus it is necessary to control dry eye and ocular surface inflammation in order to have successful surgical outcomes and to prevent recurrence in patients with pterygium.[1]

Genes associated with DNA repair, cell proliferation, migration, and angiogenesis have been shown to be associated with pterygia.[2] Chronic irritation or inflammation at the limbal area of the peripheral cornea has been suggested as the "chronic keratitis" theory, leading to focal limbal deficiency and subsequent pterygium development.[2,43,44] Human papillomavirus (HPV) has also been implicated in development.[2,45] Immunohistochemistry studies have shown the presence of six different MMPs within pterygium cells invading the cornea and may be responsible for focal destruction of Bowman's membrane.[1] These MMPs are not only capable of enzymatically degrading extracellular matrix proteins, but like other cytokines (e.g., TGF-β and IL) also play a major role in cell proliferation, migration, angiogenesis, and apoptosis.[1,2] There have also been studies of pterygia showing deregulation of TGF-β signaling and MMP overexpression, leading to increased fibroblast activity.[2,46] Increased levels of TGF-β2 in pterygia function to increase fibrotic activity; this may play an important role in pterygium pathogenesis by increasing angiogenesis and inducing differen-

tiation of pterygium fibroblasts to myofibroblasts.[47]

Successful treatment of the inflammatory aspect of ocular surface disease has been demonstrated by cyclosporine A (CsA, *Restasis*, Allergan, Dublin, Ireland). This medication has been shown to have an inhibitory effect on mRNA and protein expression of myofibroblast-related markers.[47] It has also been shown to downregulate phenotype changes of pterygium fibroblasts to TGF-β2–induced myofibroblasts.[47] The inflammatory cascade initiated by dry eye can destroy the lacrimal glands and lead to a cycle of T-cell activation and cytokine release that can damage the ocular surface, especially the conjunctival epithelium.[48] By interrupting this inflammatory cascade, the ocular surface and lacrimal gland can recover, promoting normal tear production.[48] The use of CsA has been proposed as a potential candidate for pterygium treatment, as it can inhibit fibroblast migration and MMP expression through its T-cell inactivation (and thus downstream inhibition of TGF-β2, interferon-gamma [IFN-γ], and cytokines IL-2, IL-3, and IL-4).[47]

Another study by Tong et al elaborated on the inflammatory properties of pterygia by demonstrating increased concentrations of S100 proteins on the ocular surface of these eyes.[44] The S100 proteins are calcium-binding proteins that interact with transcription factors and nucleic acids to regulate proliferation, differentiation, apoptosis, inflammation, cell migration, energy metabolism, and calcium homeostasis.[44] Specifically, S100A8 and S100A9 are involved in neutrophil chemotaxis and inflammation related to ocular surface disease (i.e., dry eye, MGD, and corneal neovascularization —all factors associated with pterygium).[44] Increased levels of S100A8 and S100A9 are present not only in ocular surface disease, but also in pterygium, at both transcriptional and protein levels.[44] The presence of these proteins in pterygia may be part of the inflammatory response of the ocular surface or response to the fibrovascularization process of pterygium growth.[44] S100A8 is induced by UV radiation, which may serve as a feedback mechanism for pterygium development.[44] As we have seen, some pterygium patients have prominent neovascular components, and that in others, the vascular component recurs after surgery, prior to the fibrous component—this may also be mediated by increased levels of S100 proteins.[44]

5.7.2 Prevention of Recurrence

Preventing pterygium recurrence is important for many reasons: patient comfort and satisfaction, decreasing patient morbidity from multiple surgeries, and the increased risk of potential dysplastic transformation of recurrent pterygia.[2,10] Although pterygia are generally considered benign lesions, many have suggested their aggressive growth patterns and growth in response to UV light exposure to be similar to certain neoplasms (e.g., squamous cell carcinoma, melanoma, and ocular surface squamous neoplasia).[10,31]

Inflammation during the postoperative period causes proliferation not only of vascular cells and fibroblasts, but also of subconjunctival fibroblast tissue and overexpression of MMPs, leading to invasive pterygia.[10] The most reliable predictor of recurrence is pterygia morphology.[10] Thick, fleshy pterygia are more likely to recur, in contrast with their atrophic counterparts (this could also explain why recurrence is more likely in younger patients, as they tend to have thicker pterygia at presentation).[10]

As mentioned earlier, inflammatory mediators such as MMPs, TGF-β2, S100 proteins, as well as feedback mechanisms present on the ocular surface (dry eye, MGD) serve as risk factors in pterygium recurrence.[10,31,42,43,44,46,47] Aggressive management of these entities is thus suggested.

5.7.3 Relationship to Neoplasia

Pterygia may have some tumor-like features, including aggressive recurrence following resection, UV radiation exposure as an etiology, and common adjunctive treatment modalities (alkylating agents and radiation).[1,2] The p53 gene has been shown to be expressed by epithelial cells in pterygia and is known to control cell differentiation, cell cycle, and apoptosis.[1] This gene is well studied and its dysregulation has been recognized in many different kinds of neoplasia that can occur throughout the body. This raises the possibility that pterygia may be a growth disorder due to uncontrolled cell proliferation, perhaps induced by p53 overexpression.[1,2]

Conjunctival intraepithelial neoplasia (CIN) contains both dysplasia and carcinoma in situ.[33] A pterygium is an invasion of the cornea with proliferation of abnormal subconjunctival tissue together with a chronic inflammatory response.[33] Carcinoma in situ has been noted to coexist in some pterygia specimen as well.[33] CIN has a close relation to pterygia as various proteins are expressed similarly in the epithelial cells of both lesions.[33] Both CIN and pterygia are associated with viral infection (e.g., HPV) and UV light exposure.[33] Of note, one report cited the incidence of CIN in pterygia to be 2.33%.[34] Thus, it is imperative to send excised pterygium specimen for histopathologic analysis and to provide long-term follow-up of these patients.[1,33] An example of a lesion referred that was thought to be an irregular pterygium, but was in fact neoplastic is shown in ▶ Fig. 5.16.

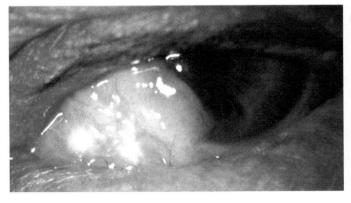

Fig. 5.16 Neoplastic lesion referred for "pterygium excision."

5.8 Conclusion

There are multiple inflammatory mediators on the macro- and micro-scale, that contribute both physiologically and structurally not only to the health of the ocular surface, but also to pterygium growth and formation. Thus, in addition to good surgical technique, it is important to aggressively manage and treat ocular surface disease (tear film deficiency, mucin deficiency, MGD, and blepharitis) in order to successfully manage these patients. The aforementioned mediators—UV exposure, disruption of tear regularity, inflammatory cytokines, and proteins (TGF-B, S100 proteins, etc.)—serve as important treatment targets both pre- and postoperatively.

References

[1] Reidy J. Corneal dystrophies, ectatic disorders and degenerations: pterygium. In: Holland E, Mannis M, eds. Cornea: Fundamentals, Diagnosis and Management. New York, NY: Elsevier; 2017:870–871

[2] Tan D, Chong E. Management of pterygium. In: Holland E, Mannis M, eds. Cornea: Surgery of the Cornea and Conjunctiva. New York, NY: Elsevier; 2017:1560–1570

[3] Anandam V. Management of pterygium. AECS Illumination.. 2015; 15(1):1–11

[4] Hirst LW. Recurrent pterygium surgery using pterygium extended removal followed by extended conjunctival transplant: recurrence rate and cosmesis. Ophthalmology. 2009; 116(7):1278–1286

[5] Prajna NV, Devi L, Seeniraj SK, Keenan JD. Conjunctival autograft versus amniotic membrane transplantation after double pterygium excision: a randomized trial. Cornea. 2016; 35(6): 823–826

[6] Clearfield E, Muthappan V, Wang X, Kuo IC. Conjunctival autograft for pterygium. The Cochrane database of systematic reviews. 2016;2:CD011349. doi:10.1002/14651858. CD011349.pub2

[7] Bloom AH, Perry HD, Donnenfeld ED, Pinchoff BS, Solomon R. Childhood onset of pterygia in twins. Eye Contact Lens. 2005; 31(6):279–280

[8] Noureddin GS, Yeung SN. The use of dry amniotic membrane in pterygium surgery. Clin Ophthalmol. 2016; 10:705–712

[9] Khan FA, Awais M, Niazi ShP, Akhter N, Ishaq M. Effectiveness of preoperative subconjunctival injection of mitomycin-C in primary pterygium surgery. J Coll Physicians Surg Pak. 2017; 27(2):88–91

[10] Nadarajah G, Ratnalingam VH, Mohd Isa H. Autologous blood versus fibrin glue in pterygium excision with conjunctival autograft surgery. Cornea. 2017; 36(4):452–456

[11] Marsit N, Gafud N, Kafou I, et al. Safety and efficacy of human amniotic membrane in primary pterygium surgery. Cell Tissue Bank. 2016; 17(3):407–412

[12] Duman F, Kosker M. Surgical management of double-head pterygium using a modified split-conjunctival autograft technique. Semin Ophthalmol. 2017; 32(6):569–574

[13] Mak RK, Chan TC, Marcet MM, et al. Use of anti-vascular endothelial growth factor in the management of pterygium. Acta Ophthalmol. 2017; 95(1):20–27

[14] Bekibele CO, Sarimiye TF, Ogundipe A, Olaniyan S. 5-Fluorouracil vs avastin as adjunct to conjunctival autograft in the surgical treatment of pterygium. Eye (Lond). 2016; 30(4): 515–521

[15] Duman F, Köşker M. Demographics of patients with double-headed pterygium and surgical outcomes. Turk J Ophthalmol. 2015; 45(6):249–253

[16] Hirst LW. Prospective study of primary pterygium surgery using pterygium extended removal followed by extended conjunctival transplantation. Ophthalmology. 2008; 115(10): 1663–1672

[17] Donnenfeld ED, Perry HD, Fromer S, Doshi S, Solomon R, Biser S. Subconjunctival mitomycin C as adjunctive therapy before pterygium excision. Ophthalmology. 2003; 110(5): 1012–1016

[18] Kampitak K, Leelawongtawun W, Leeamornsiri S, Suphacheraphan W. Role of artificial tears in reducing the recurrence of pterygium after surgery: a prospective randomized controlled trial. Acta Ophthalmol. 2017; 95: e227-e229

[19] Chaidaroon W, Pongmoragot N. Basic tear secretion measurement in pterygium. J Med Assoc Thai. 2003; 86(4):348–352

[20] Balogun MM, Ashaye AO, Ajayi BG, Osuntokun OO. Tear break-up time in eyes with pterygia and pingueculae in Ibadan. West Afr J Med. 2005; 24(2):162–166

[21] Li M, Zhang M, Lin Y, et al. Tear function and goblet cell density after pterygium excision. Eye (Lond). 2007; 21(2):224–228

[22] Julio G, Lluch S, Pujol P, Alonso S, Merindano D. Tear osmolarity and ocular changes in pterygium. Cornea. 2012; 31(12): 1417–1421

[23] Roka N, Shrestha SP, Joshi ND. Assessment of tear secretion and tear film instability in cases with pterygium and normal subjects. Nepal J Ophthalmol. 2013; 5(1):16–23

[24] Kampitak K, Leelawongtawun W. Precorneal tear film in pterygium eye. J Med Assoc Thai. 2014; 97(5):536–539

[25] Ozsutcu M, Arslan B, Erdur SK, Gulkilik G, Kocabora SM, Muftuoglu O. Tear osmolarity and tear film parameters in patients with unilateral pterygium. Cornea. 2014; 33(11): 1174–1178

[26] Kenyon KR, Wagoner MD, Hettinger ME. Conjunctival autograft transplantation for advanced and recurrent pterygium. Ophthalmology. 1985; 92(11):1461–1470

[27] Huang Y, He H, Sheha H, Tseng SC. Ocular demodicosis as a risk factor of pterygium recurrence. Ophthalmology. 2013; 120(7):1341–1347

[28] Wu H, Lin Z, Yang F, et al. Meibomian Gland Dysfunction Correlates to the Tear Film Instability and Ocular Discomfort in Patients with Pterygium. Scientific Reports. 2017;7:45115. doi:10.1038/srep45115

[29] Rajiv, Mithal S, Sood AK. Pterygium and dry eye–a clinical correlation. Indian J Ophthalmol. 1991; 39(1):15–16

[30] Ishioka M, Shimmura S, Yagi Y, Tsubota K. Pterygium and dry eye. Ophthalmologica. 2001; 215(3):209–211

[31] Folberg R. 2010. Pinguecula and Pterygium. In Kumar V, Abbas A, Fausto N, Aster J (Eds). Robbins and Cotran Pathologic Basis of Disease 8/E (pp 1349). Philadephia, PA. Saunders, an imprint of Elsevier

[32] Tan DT, Chee SP, Dear KB, Lim AS. Effect of pterygium morphology on pterygium recurrence in a controlled trial comparing conjunctival autografting with bare sclera excision. Arch Ophthalmol. 1997; 115(10):1235–1240

[33] Endo H, Kase S, Suzuki Y, Kase M. Coincidence of inflamed conjunctival carcinoma in situ and primary pterygium. Case Rep Ophthalmol. 2016; 7(3):208–212

[34] Zoroquiain P, Jabbour S, Aldrees S, et al. High frequency of squamous intraepithelial neoplasia in pterygium related to low ultraviolet light exposure. Saudi J Ophthalmol. 2016; 30 (2):113–116

[35] Shaw EL. A modified technique for conjunctival transplant. CLAO J. 1992; 18(2):112–116

[36] Kinoshita S, Friend J, Thoft RA. Ocular surface epithelial regeneration and disease. Int Ophthalmol Clin. 1984; 24(2): 169–177

[37] Hirst LW, Smallcombe K. Double-headed pterygia treated with P.E.R.F.E.C.T for pterygium. Cornea. 2017; 36(1):98–100

[38] Hovanesian JA, Starr CE, Vroman DT, et al. ASCRS Cornea Clinical Committee. Surgical techniques and adjuvants for the management of primary and recurrent pterygia. J Cataract Refract Surg. 2017; 43(3):405–419

[39] Arman A, Demirseren DD, Takmaz T. Treatment of ocular rosacea: comparative study of topical cyclosporine and oral doxycycline. Int J Ophthalmol. 2015; 8(3):544–549

[40] Rynerson JM, Perry HD. DEBS - a unification theory for dry eye and blepharitis. Clin Ophthalmol. 2016; 10(10):2455–2467

[41] Kim BY, Riaz KM, Bakhtiari P, et al. Medically reversible limbal stem cell disease: clinical features and management strategies. Ophthalmology. 2014; 121(10):2053–2058

[42] Tong L, Lan W, Sim HS, Hou A. Conjunctivochalasis is the precursor to pterygium. Med Hypotheses. 2013; 81(5): 927–930

[43] Coroneo MT, Di Girolamo N, Wakefield D. The pathogenesis of pterygia. Curr Opin Ophthalmol. 1999; 10(4):282–288

[44] Tong L, Lan W, Lim RR, Chaurasia SS. S100A proteins as molecular targets in the ocular surface inflammatory diseases. Ocul Surf. 2014; 12(1):23–31

[45] Gallagher MJ, Giannoudis A, Herrington CS, Hiscott P. Human papillomavirus in pterygium. Br J Ophthalmol. 2001; 85(7): 782–784

[46] Strong B, Farley W, Stern ME, Pflugfelder SC. Topical cyclosporine inhibits conjunctival epithelial apoptosis in experimental murine keratoconjunctivitis sicca. Cornea. 2005; 24 (1):80–85

[47] Gum SI, Kim YH, Jung JC, et al. Cyclosporine A inhibits TGF-β2-induced myofibroblasts of primary cultured human pterygium fibroblasts. Biochem Biophys Res Commun. 2017; 482(4):1148–1153

[48] Abelson M, Casavant J. Give dry eye a one-two punch. Review of ophthalmology. 2003. Available at: https://www.reviewofophthalmology.com/article/give-dry-eye-a-one-two-punch

6 Amniotic Membrane and Umbilical Cord as Platform Technology to Promote Regenerative Healing

Anny M.S. Cheng and Scheffer C.G. Tseng

Abstract

In ophthalmology, although transplanting limbal epithelial stem cells (SCs) is effective in restoring vision in eyes suffering from limbal SC deficiency, its success is threatened by nonresolving inflammation in the limbal stroma. Amniotic membrane (AM) transplantation is reintroduced to augment the success of transplantation of limbal epithelial SCs by reducing inflammation and scarring in the limbal stroma and by promoting epithelial growth. Our cumulative research effort has led to the discovery of heavy chain-hyaluronan/pentraxin 3 (HC-HA/PTX3) as one key matrix component responsible for the aforementioned therapeutic actions of AM and umbilical cord (UC). HC-HA/PTX3 is a complex formed by PTX3 tightly with HC-HA of which HA is covalently linked with HC1 derived from inter-α-trypsin inhibitor (IαI) through the catalytic action of tumor necrosis factor-stimulated gene-6 (TSG-6). Besides exerting a broad and extensive anti-inflammatory, anti-scarring, and anti-angiogenic effects, HC-HA/PTX3 also acts as "top soil" to uniquely support the phenotype of niche cells to maintain SC quiescence and retains a multi-potent plasticity of generating progenitors cells or mesenchymal SCs so as to support tissue homeostasis and regeneration. We thus envision that HC-HA/PTX3-containing therapeutics can be formulated from this platform technology to mitigate nonresolving inflammation and reinforce the well-being of SC niches beyond ophthalmology to promote regenerative healing.

Keywords: anti-inflammation, amniotic membrane, anti-scarring, Hyaluronan, Quiescence, regenerative healing, stem cell niche, umbilical cord

6.1 Introduction

Stem cells (SC) with extensive proliferative potential for giving rise to one or more differentiated cell types hold considerable promise for the treatment of a number of diseases in regenerative medicine. SCs are common in early mammalian embryos, but by adulthood, they are dispersed and kept in a unique microenvironment termed "niche" where they continue to maintain quiescence while performing relentless self-renewal to replenish the SC pool that is depleted by differentiation for the fate decision.

Among all adult epithelial tissues, the model of the corneal epithelium is most unique in its ready access and clear anatomic separation from the surrounding conjunctiva. The seminal discovery made by Dr. Tung-Tien Sun in 1986[1] taught us that corneal epithelial SCs are located at the basal epithelial layer of the limbus, which marks the junction between the cornea and the conjunctiva. Since then, cumulative studies have led us to conclude that these limbal SCs govern the homeostasis of the corneal epithelium.[1,2] This important discovery has also allowed us to use impression cytology to identify a diseased state termed "limbal SC deficiency" (LSCD) in a number of ocular surface diseases with the hallmark of "conjunctivalization" of the corneal surface.[3] Histopathologically, these diseases with LSCD also manifest superficial neovascularization, chronic stromal inflammation, and scarring.[2] Because corneal blindness caused by LSCD is due to the loss of limbal SCs, visual rehabilitation cannot be achieved by conventional corneal transplantation. Hence, the aforementioned discovery has also led us to devise transplantation of autologous limbal SCs in 1989 for unilateral LSCD[4] and transplantation of allogeneic limbal SCs in 1994 for bilateral LSCD.[5] Although many subsequent studies have confirmed their clinical efficacy in patients with LSCD, one case with acute chemical burn was noted to have unsatisfactory outcome as early as 1989 when transplantation of autologous limbal SCs was first reported.[4] Late on, we then identified nonresolving inflammation in the limbal stroma as a likely cause of failure in an experimental rabbit model of LSCD caused by a combination of chemical and mechanical insults.[6]

To examine the hypothesis that severely or chronically inflamed limbal stroma is not suitable for receiving transplanted limbal SCs, we then sought for a means to restore a healthy and supportive limbal stromal niche. Therefore, we tested transplantation of human amniotic membrane (AM) and reported in 1995 that this surgical procedure alone can restore a normal corneal surface in 5 (38%) of 13 rabbits when compared to 0 (0%) of

10 untransplanted rabbits that suffered from acute chemical burns.[7] To draw a plausible relationship between AM transplantation (AMT) and limbal SC transplantation, we proposed in 1997 a metaphor, in which the former serves as "top soil" to support the latter, which acts as if we plant the "seed" in a garden.[8] This hypothetical viewpoint has since been substantiated by a number of clinical studies. For example, AMT alone can prevent LSCD in acute chemical burns[9,10] and acute Stevens–Johnson syndrome[11,12,13] to restore vision in corneas with partial (i.e., < 360° involvement) LSCD[14,15] and to augment the success of transplanting autologous[16,17] and allogeneic[5,18] limbal SCs for corneas with total LSCD. Furthermore, AM as a single[19] and dual layers[20] is also used to aid in vivo expansion of limbal SCs in a new surgical procedure termed "simple limbal epithelial transplantation" as well as used as a substrate or carrier to promote ex vivo expansion of limbal SCs.[21]

6.2 Clinical Ophthalmic Indications

Since our first reintroduction of AMT in 1995 in ophthalmology,[7] over 1,000 peer-reviewed publications have been published in the last 20 years describing the clinical efficacies of AMT for treating diverse ocular surface diseases. In 2001, through a formal process of Request for Designation, the U.S. Food and Drug Administration (FDA) ruled that transplantation of cryopreserved human AM (manufactured by Bio-Tissue, Inc.) for ocular surface reconstruction is classified as "361 human cell/tissue products (HCT/P)" to exert anti-inflammatory, anti-scarring, and anti-angiogenic actions to promote wound healing. Subsequently, the Centers of Medicare and Medicaid Services (CMS) in the United States of America has granted three level 1 CPT codes to cover the surgical procedures of transplanting cryopreserved AM and umbilical cord (UC) for a number of ophthalmic indications (▶ Fig. 6.1).

In brief, these indications can be categorized into the following two modes of AMT, that is, as a graft and as a biological bandage (▶ Fig. 6.1).[22] Intuitively, when AMT is used as a graft, it is meant to fill in the tissue defect. Upon healing, the membrane is integrated into the host tissue as host cells grow over or into the membrane to restore the tissue integrity and function. In this mode, AM can be used as a single or multiple layers and secured

to the host tissue by sutures or fibrin glue in a sutureless manner. In the second mode, AM is used as a bandage to cover both the site of interest and the healthy host tissue at the same time by sutures or via placement of "sutureless" ProKera (Bio-Tissue, Inc., Miami, FL). This mode is usually considered when there is no/minimal stromal loss and the host epithelium heals underneath the membrane.

ProKera is classified as a type II medical device by the FDA via 510(k) clearance and contains a polycarbonate ring system that fastens cryopreserved AM in between. The sutureless approach via ProKera shortens the surgical time, permits topical anesthesia, and eliminates suture-induced inflammation. It can be applied in the office, the emergency room, and the hospital bedside to facilitate "early intervention" and reduces the overall medical cost. This is particularly important for managing acute chemical burns[9,10] and acute Stevens–Johnson syndrome/toxic epidermal necrolysis[11,12,13] that require acute intervention. Upon healing, ProKera can be removed in the practitioner's office. If the AM dissolves sooner than expected, one may like to look into "exposure" issue caused by infrequent blinking with incomplete closure. In this regard, ProKera may facilitate blinking because of the polycarbonate ring. This likelihood is supported by accelerated restoration of the corneal surface not only in the eye with the placement of ProKera but sometimes also in the fellow eye without.[23] Occasionally, AM can be used as both a graft and a patch in one patient to further augment the therapeutic benefit of the transplanted AM graft.[14,20] Self-retained AM also may attract inflammatory cells out of the ocular surface, become cloudy, lose its potency, and may require replacement to achieve continuous effectiveness.

6.3 Mechanism of Action of Amniotic Membrane and Umbilical Cord

The aforementioned clinical efficacies observed in ophthalmology let us wonder what can be the underlying mechanism of action cryopreserved AM/UC. Anatomically, the AM is the innermost membrane enwrapping the fetus in the amniotic cavity and extends from the fetal membrane to the UC. Developmentally, both the AM and UC share the same cell origin as the fetus. The traditional

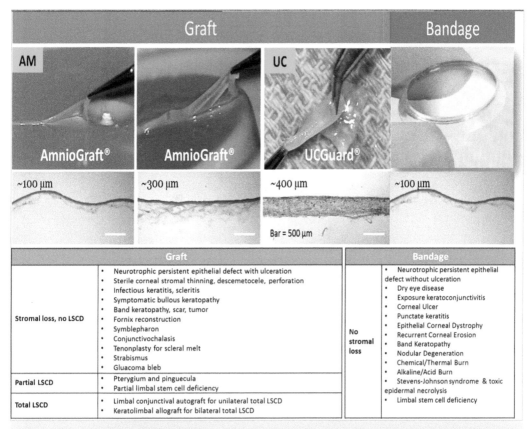

	Graft		Bandage
Stromal loss, no LSCD	• Neurotrophic persistent epithelial defect with ulceration • Sterile corneal stromal thinning, descemetocele, perforation • Infectious keratitis, scleritis • Symptomatic bullous keratopathy • Band keratopathy, scar, tumor • Fornix reconstruction • Symblepharon • Conjunctivochalasis • Tenonplasty for scleral melt • Strabismus • Gluacoma bleb	No stromal loss	• Neurotrophic persistent epithelial defect without ulceration • Dry eye disease • Exposure keratoconjunctivitis • Corneal Ulcer • Punctate keratitis • Epithelial Corneal Dystrophy • Recurrent Corneal Erosion • Band Keratopathy • Nodular Degeneration • Chemical/Thermal Burn • Alkaline/Acid Burn • Stevens-Johnson syndrome & toxic epidermal necrolysis
Partial LSCD	• Pterygium and pinguecula • Partial limbal stem cell deficiency		• Limbal stem cell deficiency
Total LSCD	• Limbal conjunctival autograft for unilateral total LSCD • Keratolimbal allograft for bilateral total LSCD		

Fig. 6.1 Clinical ophthalmic indications. AM or UC can be used as a permanent surgical graft or temporary bandage. When there is stromal loss but no LSCD, AM/UC is used as a permanent graft to fill in the tissue defect for the host cells to grow and to restore the tissue integrity and function. When partial LSCD is involved, AM/UC is an effective approach to expand the preserved SC pool. Additionally, AM/UC can augment the success of transplanting limbal SCs in total LSCD. AM via placement of "sutureless" ProKera can be used as a temporary biological bandage to reduce inflammation and scarring and to promote epithelial healing when there is no/minimal stromal loss in the corneal stroma. AM, amniotic membrane; LSCD, limbal stem cell deficiency; SC, stem cell; UC, umbilical cord.

view of AM and UC is their protective function of the fetus during pregnancy. However, the fact that AM/UC can serve as a graft and as a bandage strongly suggests that this birth tissue can be a "structural" scaffold (as a graft) as well as a "biological" bandage. It also suggests that the biological factor(s) in this birth tissue may be releasable from the tissue to exert colossal anti-inflammatory, anti-scarring, and anti-angiogenic actions.

To search for the relevant biological characteristic of these birth tissues, we have embarked on a 12-year journey from 2002 to 2014. We first verified that the aforementioned anti-inflammatory action exerted by cryopreserved AM is retained in the water-soluble AM extract (AME) prepared from cryopreserved AM. Specifically, we have

shown that human AME can induce apoptosis of IFN-γ, lipopolysaccharide (LPS), and IFN-γ/LPS-activated, but not resting macrophages.[24,25] AME also downregulates expression of M1 macrophage markers, such as TNF-α, IL-6, CD86, and MHC II while upregulating M2 macrophage markers such as cytokine IL-10.[25]

Following the work of identifying the HC-HA/PTX3 complex as the key component in the cumulus-oocyte complex surrounding the ovulated oocyte to ensure fertilization,[26,27] our laboratory was the first reporting that the same biosynthetic pathway used for ovulation also takes place in the AM. In short, we have purified the HC-HA/PTX3 complex from AME by two successive runs of ultracentrifugation in a cesium chloride (CsCl)

Step 1

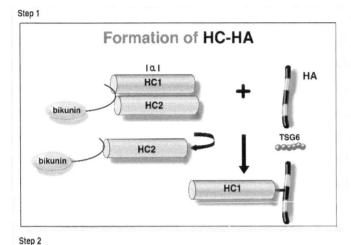

Formation of **HC-HA**

Step 2

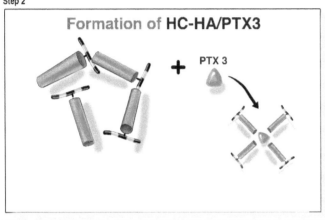

Formation of **HC-HA/PTX3**

Fig. 6.2 Formation of the key novel matrix component, HC-HA/PTX3, in AM and UC. The HC-HA/PTX3 is responsible for AM's therapeutic actions[28,29] and is found in the UC at significantly greater quantities.[30] IαI is composed of two HCs (HC1 and HC2) covalently linked to bikunin via a chondroitin sulfate. HCs from IαI are covalently transferred to HMW HA to form HC–HA complex via the catalytic action of TSG-6. PTX3 octamers are tightly associated with the HC–HA complex via binding with HCs. AM, amniotic membrane; HA, hyaluronan; HC, heavy chain; IαI, inter-α-trypsin inhibitor; PTX3, pentraxin 3; TSG-6, tumor necrosis factor-stimulated gene-6; UC, umbilical cord. (Reproduced with permission from Guan and Tseng.[31])

gradient in the presence of 4 M guanidine hydrochloride (HCl).[28,29] The biosynthetic process of HC-HA/PTX3 involves two steps (▶ Fig. 6.2): the first is to form HCHA complex via the catalytic action of tumor necrosis factor-stimulated gene-6 (TSG-6) resulting in the covalent (ester bond) transfer of HC1 from inter-α-trypsin inhibitor (IαI) to high molecular weight HA (> 3,000 kDa). The source of IαI, which contains two HCs (i.e., HC1 and HC2) and a light chain termed bikunin, is the serum following secretion from the liver for ovulation. However, we discovered that IαI is endogenously produced by AM epithelial cells and stromal cells to circumvent the shortcoming of this avascular tissue. The expression of TSG-6 and PTX3 is constitutive (i.e., without relying on proinflammatory cytokines). The second step is to form the HC-HA/PTX complex by tight association of the HC-HA complex with PTX3.

6.3.1 Anti-inflammatory, Anti-scarring, and Anti-angiogenic effect of HC-HA/PTX3

In contrast to HA, HC-HA/PTX3 significantly promotes apoptosis of activated but not resting polymorphonuclear neutrophils (PMNs) and macrophages. In addition, HC-HA/PTX3 promotes phagocytosis of apoptotic PMNs by resting and activated macrophages.[32] Therefore, HC-HA/PTX3 suppresses proinflammatory responses of neutrophils and macrophages involved in innate immune responses. Furthermore, HC-HA/PTX3 promotes polarization of activated macrophages toward M2 phenotype, which express a high level of anti-inflammatory IL-10, to activate Treg lymphocytes that result in downregulation of inflammatory response by Th1 and Th17 lymphocytes.[32] Given that macrophages are at the cross-road bridging innate immune responses and adaptive immune responses, the anti-inflammatory effect of HC-HA/PTX3 in innate immune responses is also extended to modulate adaptive immune responses[33] to gear pathological wound healing toward regeneration. The HC-HA/PTX3 has not only indirect anti-scarring effects from anti-inflammatory responses but also a direct anti-scarring effect. This direct anti-scarring effect is evidenced by the reduction of myofibroblast differentiation with AM implantation[34] and reduction of corneal haze in excimer laser-induced keratectomy in rabbits.[35] Recent study has shown that HC-HA/PTX3 suppresses the TGFβ1 promoter activity of human corneal fibroblasts.[32] Besides reduction of inflammation and scarring, AMT corneal surfaces also show reduced vascularization.[36] HC-HA/PTX3 suppresses human umbilical vascular endothelial cells (HUVEC) viability, inhibits proliferation, and causes HUVEC to become small and rounded with a decrease in spreading and filamentous actin.[37] Migration triggered by VEGF and tube formation was also significantly inhibited by HC-HA/PTX3.[37]

6.3.2 HC-HA/PTX3 Maintains Limbal Niche Cell Phenotype for Supporting SC Quiescence

Successful isolation and expansion of limbal niche cells (LNCs)[38,39] has allowed us to establish an in vitro model of sphere growth generated by reunion between limbal epithelial progenitor cells (LEPCs) and expanded LNCs. The close contact of LEPCs with LNCs prevents corneal epithelial differentiation.[39,40] Both bone morphogenetic protein (BMP) and Wnt signaling control SCs in various epithelial tissues. Under immobilized HC-HA/PTX3, the resultant spheres of LEPCs and LNCs upregulate quiescence markers, but negligible clonal growth of LEPCs.[41] This outcome was correlated with the suppression of canonical Wnt, but activation of noncanonical (planar cell polarity [PCP]) Wnt signaling as well as BMP signaling in both LEPCs and LNCs. HC-HA/PTX3 uniquely upregulates BMP signaling in LNCs, which leads to BMP signaling in LEPCs to achieve quiescence. This finding helps explain how AMT is clinically useful as a matrix for both in vivo[19] and ex vivo[21] expansion of limbal epithelial SCs and to treat corneal blindness caused by LSCD.

6.4 Platform Technology: Clinical Applications beyond Ophthalmology

Adult wound healing is heralded by inflammation, which involve cellular infiltration by PMNs, macrophages, and lymphocytes derived from innate and adaptive immune responses, respectively. PMNs are among the first recruited to engulf pathogens and damaged tissues before their eventual apoptosis. These apoptotic PMNs are phagocytized by M2 macrophages to restore and maintain anti-inflammatory and immune-tolerogenic milieu.[42] On the contrary, under pathological states, PMNs delay apoptosis to exacerbate inflammation and activate M1 macrophages that are ineffective in phagocytic clearance of apoptotic PMN.[43] M1 macrophages are also professed to activate Th1 and Th17 lymphocytes that play a key role in allogeneic rejection and autoimmune dysregulation, respectively. A lack of transition from M1 to M2 macrophages is a hallmark of nonhealing skin wounds. Collectively, these pathological states lead to prolonged inflammation that is the hallmark of a number of diseases.[44,45]

As a contrast, fetal wound healing is characterized as "scarless."[46,47] The inflammatory response (by virtue of a less than mature immune system) in the fetus is less pronounced and differs from the postnatal state in the types and number of inflammatory cells that enter the wound.[48,49,50] Besides downregulation of pro-inflammatory responses, a downregulation of pro-scarring response in fetal wound healing occurs.[51,52] The aforementioned molecular mechanism of HC-HA/PTX3 suggests that cryopreserved AM/UC delivers synergistic actions of reducing inflammation, suppressing fibrosis, and promoting epithelialization desirable for regenerative healing.[44,45] This concept was first examined in the safety and efficacy of cryopreserved UC in promoting wound healing in rats and sheep models of surgically created spina bifida. Cryopreserved UC not only completely seals the defect, prevents CSF leakage, reverses the Chiari II malformation, and preserves the spinal cord tissue,[53,54,55,56,57,58] but also regenerates skin components with minimal inflammatory cells[54] Currently, cryopreserved UC has been used during in utero repair of a large myeloschisis (a more severe form of spina bifida) in a total of four human cases with satisfactory preliminary regenerative healing

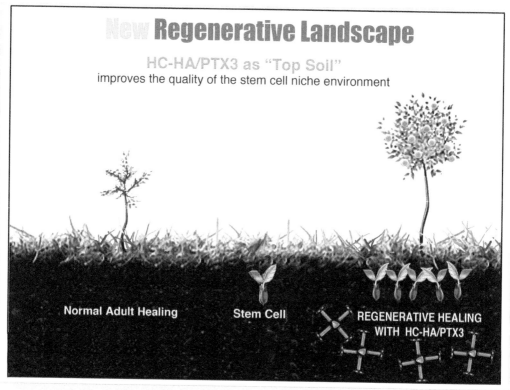

Fig. 6.3 HC-HA/PTX3 as a novel regenerative matrix. The concept that HC-HA/PTX3 as "weeding and pruning" of undesired inflammation and scarring and "nutrient supply in top soil" to improve the quality of SC niche environment is illustrated in a new landscape as a metaphor to illustrate that HC-HA/PTX3 is a novel regenerative matrix. The metaphor is modified from that first conceived in 1997[8] and by incorporating the cumulative understanding of HC-HA/PTX3 as a novel regenerative matrix.[44,45] HA, hyaluronan; HC, heavy chain; PTX3, pentraxin 3.

results. Likewise, cryopreserved UC has also been used to treat a variety of foot and ankle problems including chronic nonhealing wounds[59,60,61,62] and wounds that are complicated by exposed tendon, muscle, joint capsule, and/or bone, and with histopathological confirmation of osteomyelitis.[63] Consequently, we envision that the HCHA/PTX3 complex is a unique matrix that can be formulated as a platform technology to launch many other therapeutics beyond the ocular surface to aid regeneration in the future.

6.5 New Landscape of Regenerative Therapies Based on HC-HA/PTX3

Cumulative understanding of HC-HA/PTX3 as a novel regenerative matrix[44,45] has allowed us to repaint a new landscape of regenerative therapies

using the metaphor of growing a tree in the garden first conceived in 1997[8] (▶ Fig. 6.3). First, because nonresolving inflammation present in the host tissue is a common threat of diverse diseases and an impediment against the success of transplanted limbal epithelial SCs, we believe that HC-HA/PTX3 acts by "weeding and pruning" to effectively control inflammation and to prevent scarring. The anti-inflammatory action of HC-HA/PTX3 stands out as a unique class of biologic because it exerts broad anti-inflammatory actions by targeting PMN, macrophages, and lymphocytes from innate to adaptive immune responses. The anti-scarring action of HC-HA/PTX3 secures an appropriate matrix rigidity so that it maintains the progenitor status because an increase in matrix rigidity due to scarring threatens the SC well-being and facilitates tissue/organ failure.[64,65] Second, HC-HA/PTX3 acts as "topsoil" to support the phenotype of niche cells to secure SC quiescence that is essential to tissue homeostasis and regeneration. Because maintenance of such a phenotype of niche cells in the limbal SC niche retains a multipotent plasticity of generating angiogenesis progenitors, pericytes, and mesenchymal SCs, HC-HA/PTX3 provides a fertile ground for supporting the formation of regenerative tissues via revascularization and reinnervation. Future studies are warranted to substantiate such a new regenerative landscape.

Conflicts of Interest: Dr. Tseng is the founder and a major shareholder of TissueTech Inc., which holds patents on the methods of preservation and clinical uses of cryopreserved amniotic membrane graft, ProKera, and umbilical cord products.

Financial Disclosure: The development of Pro-Kera was supported in part with grant number EY014768 from the National Institute of Health (NIH) and National Eye Institute (NEI). The content is solely the responsibility of the authors and does not necessarily represent the opinion of the NIH or the NEI.

References

[1] Schermer A, Galvin S, Sun TT. Differentiation-related expression of a major 64K corneal keratin in vivo and in culture suggests limbal location of corneal epithelial stem cells. J Cell Biol. 1986; 103(1):49–62

[2] Lavker RM, Tseng SC, Sun TT. Corneal epithelial stem cells at the limbus: looking at some old problems from a new angle. Exp Eye Res. 2004; 78(3):433–446

[3] Puangsricharern V, Tseng SC. Cytologic evidence of corneal diseases with limbal stem cell deficiency. Ophthalmology. 1995; 102(10):1476–1485

[4] Kenyon KR, Tseng SC. Limbal autograft transplantation for ocular surface disorders. Ophthalmology. 1989; 96(5):709–722, discussion 722–723

[5] Tsai RJF, Tseng SC. Human allograft limbal transplantation for corneal surface reconstruction. Cornea. 1994; 13(5):389–400

[6] Tsai RJF, Tseng SC. Effect of stromal inflammation on the outcome of limbal transplantation for corneal surface reconstruction. Cornea. 1995; 14(5):439–449

[7] Kim JC, Tseng SC. Transplantation of preserved human amniotic membrane for surface reconstruction in severely damaged rabbit corneas. Cornea. 1995; 14(5):473–484

[8] Tseng SC, Tsubota K. Important concepts for treating ocular surface and tear disorders. Am J Ophthalmol. 1997; 124(6):825–835

[9] Kheirkhah A, Johnson DA, Paranjpe DR, Raju VK, Casas V, Tseng SC. Temporary sutureless amniotic membrane patch for acute alkaline burns. Arch Ophthalmol. 2008; 126(8):1059–1066

[10] Meller D, Pires RTF, Mack RJS, et al. Amniotic membrane transplantation for acute chemical or thermal burns. Ophthalmology. 2000; 107(5):980–989, discussion 990

[11] Gregory DG. Treatment of acute Stevens-Johnson syndrome and toxic epidermal necrolysis using amniotic membrane: a review of 10 consecutive cases. Ophthalmology. 2011; 118 (5):908–914

[12] Shammas MC, Lai EC, Sarkar JS, Yang J, Starr CE, Sippel KC. Management of acute Stevens-Johnson syndrome and toxic epidermal necrolysis utilizing amniotic membrane and topical corticosteroids. Am J Ophthalmol. 2010; 149(2):203–213.e2

[13] Fu Y, Gregory DG, Sippel KC, Bouchard CS, Tseng SC. The ophthalmologist's role in the management of acute Stevens-Johnson syndrome and toxic epidermal necrolysis. Ocul Surf. 2010; 8(4):193–203

[14] Kheirkhah A, Casas V, Raju VK, Tseng SC. Sutureless amniotic membrane transplantation for partial limbal stem cell deficiency. Am J Ophthalmol. 2008; 145(5):787–794

[15] Anderson DF, Ellies P, Pires RT, Tseng SC. Amniotic membrane transplantation for partial limbal stem cell deficiency. Br J Ophthalmol. 2001; 85(5):567–575

[16] Meallet MA, Espana EM, Grueterich M, Ti SE, Goto E, Tseng SC. Amniotic membrane transplantation with conjunctival limbal autograft for total limbal stem cell deficiency. Ophthalmology. 2003; 110(8):1585–1592

[17] Kheirkhah A, Raju VK, Tseng SC. Minimal conjunctival limbal autograft for total limbal stem cell deficiency. Cornea. 2008; 27(6):730–733

[18] Tseng SC, Prabhasawat P, Barton K, Gray T, Meller D. Amniotic membrane transplantation with or without limbal allografts for corneal surface reconstruction in patients with limbal stem cell deficiency. Arch Ophthalmol. 1998; 116(4):431–441

[19] Sangwan VS, Basu S, MacNeil S, Balasubramanian D. Simple limbal epithelial transplantation (SLET): a novel surgical technique for the treatment of unilateral limbal stem cell deficiency. Br J Ophthalmol. 2012; 96(7):931–934

[20] Amescua G, Atallah M, Nikpoor N, Galor A, Perez VL. Modified simple limbal epithelial transplantation using cryopreserved amniotic membrane for unilateral limbal stem cell deficiency. Am J Ophthalmol. 2014; 158(3):469–75.e2

[21] Tseng SC, Chen SY, Shen YC, Chen WL, Hu FR. Critical appraisal of ex vivo expansion of human limbal epithelial stem cells. Curr Mol Med. 2010; 10(9):841–850

[22] Liu J, Sheha H, Fu Y, Liang L, Tseng SC. Update on amniotic membrane transplantation. Expert Rev Ophthalmol. 2010; 5 (5):645–661

[23] Cheng AM, Zhao D, Chen R, et al. Accelerated restoration of ocular surface health in dry eye disease by self-retained cryopreserved amniotic membrane. Ocul Surf. 2016; 14(1):56–63

[24] Li W, He H, Kawakita T, Espana EM, Tseng SC. Amniotic membrane induces apoptosis of interferon-gamma activated macrophages in vitro. Exp Eye Res. 2006; 82(2):282–292

[25] He H, Li W, Chen SY, et al. Suppression of activation and induction of apoptosis in RAW264.7 cells by amniotic membrane extract. Invest Ophthalmol Vis Sci. 2008; 49(10):4468–4475

[26] Zhuo L, Yoneda M, Zhao M, et al. Defect in SHAP-hyaluronan complex causes severe female infertility. A study by inactivation of the bikunin gene in mice. J Biol Chem. 2001; 276(11):7693–7696

[27] Salustri A, Garlanda C, Hirsch E, et al. PTX3 plays a key role in the organization of the cumulus oophorus extracellular matrix and in in vivo fertilization. Development. 2004; 131 (7):1577–1586

[28] He H, Li W, Tseng DY, et al. Biochemical characterization and function of complexes formed by hyaluronan and the heavy chains of inter-alpha-inhibitor (HC*HA) purified from extracts of human amniotic membrane. J Biol Chem. 2009; 284(30):20136–20146

[29] Zhang S, He H, Day AJ, Tseng SC. Constitutive expression of inter-α-inhibitor (IαI) family proteins and tumor necrosis factor-stimulated gene-6 (TSG-6) by human amniotic membrane epithelial and stromal cells supporting formation of

the heavy chain-hyaluronan (HC-HA) complex. J Biol Chem. 2012; 287(15):12433–12444

[30] Tan EK, Cooke M, Mandrycky C, et al. Structural and biological comparison of cryopreserved and fresh amniotic membrane tissues. J Biomater Tissue Eng. 2014; 4(5): 379–388

[31] Guan Y, Tseng SC. Regenerative healing: science pointing to a cure. Pain Med.. in press

[32] He H, Zhang S, Tighe S, Son J, Tseng SC. Immobilized heavy chain-hyaluronic acid polarizes lipopolysaccharide-activated macrophages toward M2 phenotype. J Biol Chem. 2013; 288 (36):25792–25803

[33] He H, Tan Y, Duffort S, Perez VL, Tseng SC. In vivo downregulation of innate and adaptive immune responses in corneal allograft rejection by HC-HA/PTX3 complex purified from amniotic membrane. Invest Ophthalmol Vis Sci. 2014; 55(3): 1647–1656

[34] Choi TH, Tseng SC. In vivo and in vitro demonstration of epithelial cell-induced myofibroblast differentiation of keratocytes and an inhibitory effect by amniotic membrane. Cornea. 2001; 20(2):197–204

[35] Wang MX, Gray TB, Parks WC, et al. Reduction in corneal haze and apoptosis by amniotic membrane matrix in excimer laser photoablation in rabbits. J Cataract Refract Surg. 2001; 27:310–319

[36] Kim JC, Tseng SC. The effects on inhibition of corneal neovascularization after human amniotic membrane transplantation in severely damaged rabbit corneas. Korean J Ophthalmol. 1995; 9(1):32–46

[37] Shay E, Khadem JJ, Tseng SC. Efficacy and limitation of sutureless amniotic membrane transplantation for acute toxic epidermal necrolysis. Cornea. 2010; 29(3):359–361

[38] Xie HT, Chen SY, Li GG, Tseng SC. Limbal epithelial stem/progenitor cells attract stromal niche cells by SDF-1/CXCR4 signaling to prevent differentiation. Stem Cells. 2011; 29(11): 1874–1885

[39] Li GG, Chen SY, Xie HT, Zhu YT, Tseng SC. Angiogenesis potential of human limbal stromal niche cells. Invest Ophthalmol Vis Sci. 2012; 53(7):3357–3367

[40] Xie HT, Chen SY, Li GG, Tseng SC. Isolation and expansion of human limbal stromal niche cells. Invest Ophthalmol Vis Sci. 2012; 53(1):279–286

[41] Chen SY, Han B, Zhu YT, et al. HC-HA/PTX3 purified from amniotic membrane promotes BMP signaling in limbal niche cells to maintain quiescence of limbal epithelial progenitor/stem cells. Stem Cells. 2015; 33(11):3341–3355

[42] Fadok VA, Bratton DL, Konowal A, Freed PW, Westcott JY, Henson PM. Macrophages that have ingested apoptotic cells in vitro inhibit proinflammatory cytokine production through autocrine/paracrine mechanisms involving TGF-beta, PGE2, and PAF. J Clin Invest. 1998; 101(4):890–898

[43] Khanna S, Biswas S, Shang Y, et al. Macrophage dysfunction impairs resolution of inflammation in the wounds of diabetic mice. PLoS One. 2010; 5(3):e9539

[44] Tseng SC. HC-HA/PTX3 purified from amniotic membrane as novel regenerative matrix: insight into relationship between inflammation and regeneration. Invest Ophthalmol Vis Sci. 2016; 57(5):ORSFh1–8

[45] Tseng SC, He H, Zhang S, Chen SY. Niche regulation of limbal epithelial stem cells: relationship between inflammation and regeneration. Ocul Surf. 2016; 14(2):100–112

[46] Rolfe KJ, Grobbelaar AO. A review of fetal scarless healing. ISRN Dermatol. 2012; 2012:698034

[47] Larson BJ, Longaker MT, Lorenz HP. Scarless fetal wound healing: a basic science review. Plast Reconstr Surg. 2010; 126 (4):1172–1180

[48] Cowin AJ, Holmes TM, Brosnan P, Ferguson MW. Expression of TGF-beta and its receptors in murine fetal and adult dermal wounds. Eur J Dermatol. 2001; 11(5):424–431

[49] Liechty KW, Adzick NS, Crombleholme TM. Diminished interleukin 6 (IL-6) production during scarless human fetal wound repair. Cytokine. 2000; 12(6):671–676

[50] Liechty KW, Crombleholme TM, Cass DL, Martin B, Adzick NS. Diminished interleukin-8 (IL-8) production in the fetal wound healing response. J Surg Res. 1998; 77(1):80–84

[51] Sullivan KM, Lorenz HP, Meuli M, Lin RY, Adzick NS. A model of scarless human fetal wound repair is deficient in transforming growth factor beta. J Pediatr Surg. 1995; 30(2):198–202, discussion 202–203

[52] Olutoye OO, Yager DR, Cohen IK, Diegelmann RF. Lower cytokine release by fetal porcine platelets: a possible explanation for reduced inflammation after fetal wounding. J Pediatr Surg. 1996; 31(1):91–95

[53] Papanna R, Mann LK, Snowise S, et al. Neurological outcomes after human umbilical cord patch for in utero spina bifida repair in a sheep model. AJP Rep. 2016; 6(3):e309–e317

[54] Papanna R, Moise KJ , Jr, Mann LK, et al. Cryopreserved human umbilical cord patch for in-utero spina bifida repair. Ultrasound Obstet Gynecol. 2016; 47(2):168–176

[55] Papanna R, Mann LK, Tseng SC, et al. Cryopreserved human amniotic membrane and a bioinspired underwater adhesive to seal and promote healing of iatrogenic fetal membrane defect sites. Placenta. 2015; 36(8):888–894

[56] Papanna R, Mann L, Fletcher S, et al. Cryopreserved human umbilical cord (HUC) as a regenerative patch material for in-utero repair of myelomeningocele (MMC) to preserve neuronal anatomy. Am J Obstet Gynecol. 2015; 212(1):S46–S47

[57] Papanna R, Mann LK, Won JH, et al. Conventional vs cryopreserved human umbilical cord (HUC) patch based repair for in-utero spina bifida in a sheep model. Am J Obstet Gynecol. 2017; 216(1):S61–S62

[58] Mann LK, Won JH, Snowise S, et al. Cryopreserved human umbilical cord (HUC) vs acellular dermal matrix (ADM) for in-utero spina bifida repair. Am J Obstet Gynecol. 2017; 216 (1):S60–S61

[59] Chua LSM, O'Connell J, Kang S, et al. An open label prospective pilot study to evaluate the efficacy of cryopreserved amniotic tissue grafts for chronic non-healing ulcers. Wounds. 2014; 26(5):E30–E38

[60] DeMill SL, Granata JD, McAlister JE, Berlet GC, Hyer CF. Safety analysis of cryopreserved amniotic membrane/umbilical cord tissue in foot and ankle surgery: a consecutive case series of 124 patients. Surg Technol Int. 2014; 25:257–261

[61] Ellington JK, Ferguson CM. The use of amniotic membrane/umbilical cord in first metatarsophalangeal joint cheilectomy: a comparative bilateral case study. Surg Technol Int. 2014; 25:63–67

[62] Warner M, Lasyone L. An open-label, single-center, retrospective study of cryopreserved amniotic membrane and umbilical cord tissue as an adjunct for foot and ankle surgery. Surg Technol Int. 2014; 25:251–255

[63] Caputo WJ, Vaquero C, Monterosa A, et al. A retrospective study of cryopreserved umbilical cord as an adjunctive therapy to promote the healing of chronic, complex foot ulcers with underlying osteomyelitis. Wound Repair Regen. 2016; 24(5):885–893

[64] Huang NF, Li S. Regulation of the matrix microenvironment for stem cell engineering and regenerative medicine. Ann Biomed Eng. 2011; 39(4):1201–1214

[65] Liu WF. Mechanical regulation of cellular phenotype: implications for vascular tissue regeneration. Cardiovasc Res. 2012; 95(2):215–222

7 Conjunctival Autograft for Primary and Recurrent Pterygium: Past, Present, and Future

Minas T. Coroneo

Abstract

A key to the success of gold standard pterygium surgery is the construction and management of conjunctival/limbal-conjunctival autografts. This technique is associated with relatively low recurrence and complication rates as well as excellent cosmesis. A core concept is that this procedure is reconstructive in contradistinction to the destructive procedures that are often still used. The evolution of these surgical techniques is traced from early success with the use of skin and mucous membrane grafts to the current method, described in the 1930s and to present day femtosecond laser-assisted conjunctival flaps (FLAPS). These techniques allow wide excision of chronically inflamed tissue, reducing the risk of leaving behind unsuspected neoplasia as well as the risk of inflammatory mediator-induced "pseudo" dry eye syndrome. Healing can proceed by primary intention with minimal scarring, providing a better functional and cosmetic result. As a consequence of very low recurrence rates, intervention can now be proposed early in the course of the disease, thereby minimizing the risk of sight-blunting sequelae, such as corneal extension and significant astigmatism. The author's current technique is described in detail, and the management of ocular surface inflammation is emphasized. Novel insights into risk factors for graft failure are described as well as the use of hyperbaric oxygen to support at-risk grafts in cases previously exposed to radiation, mitomycin C (MMC), or vascular endothelial growth factor (VEGF) inhibitors. Since pterygium can have high prevalence in some communities, teaching of this procedure to novice surgeons is discussed.

Keywords: pterygium, surgery, autoconjunctival graft, limbal-autoconjunctival, recurrence rate, femtosecond laser, dry eye, cosmesis, astigmatism

7.1 Introduction

Pterygium, a prevalent ophthalmic Cinderella disease, has consequences for the eye, patient, and community that are often underestimated.[1] Sometimes trivialized as a minor ailment, advances in our understanding of the basic pathophysiology of this condition as well as refinement of surgical techniques have resulted in improved outcomes.[2,3,4] Central to this pterygium surgery renaissance has been the use of a reconstructive rather than a destructive surgical approach through the use of conjunctival (CAG) and limbal-conjunctival autografting (LCAG).[2] This chapter will trace the history of the evolution of these procedures and examine the reasons for their success. Further refinement of these techniques will also be explored.

7.2 Background

The mission in pterygium surgery is to restore ocular surface anatomy, function, and cosmesis both in the short and long term and in so doing, alleviate all associated symptoms, painlessly and cost effectively. The plethora of surgical techniques utilized[2] to achieve these ends is evidence of both lack of deep understanding of the pathophysiology of this disease[2,3,4,5] and until recent times, lack of evidence of superiority of a particular intervention.

Pterygium surgery has evolved through a number of eras with the possibility of

- Minimal recurrence.
- Ocular surface rehabilitation.
- Excellent cosmesis.
- Minimal refractive error.

This has contributed to a shift toward earlier intervention with an aim of keeping induced corneal astigmatism to less than 0.5D, a level at which there is minimal effect on visual acuity and later in life,[6] to allow the maximal benefit of high quality intraocular lenses. This may be of particular importance since there is an association between the presence of pterygium and cataract.[7]

Pterygium impacts quality of life, affecting the psyche (redness and dryness), blunting sight via several mechanisms and can result in blindness via transcorneal extension.[2] It can threaten the eye (largely as a consequence of adjunctive measures, such as mitomycin C [MMC]) with subsequent infection and can threaten life if a diagnosis of malignancy, such as mucoepidermoid or squamous spindle cell carcinoma, is missed.[8,9]

CAG/LCAGs address these issues. Thin, Tenon's free, adequately sized, tension-free grafts tend not to retract and are associated with good outcomes.[2,10] They allow wide pterygium excision so that chronically inflamed pterygium tissue (a source of inflammatory mediators) is removed, reducing the risk of a "pseudo" dry eye state seen in pterygium patients.[11] Wide excision also results in a better cosmetic result[2,12,13] and also reduces the risk of leaving behind ocular surface squamous neoplasia (OSSN) that can occur in ~ 10 to 30% of pterygia[14,15] and atypical epithelial and melanocytic lesions in 12% of pterygia.[14,16]

Very low recurrence rates (< 1%) have been reported for this approach despite varying excision techniques.[2,17,18] Recently a Cochrane meta-analysis demonstrated that conjunctival autograft is associated with a lower risk of recurrence at 6 months after surgery than amniotic membrane transplantation.[19] Furthermore patients with recurrent pterygia had a lower risk of recurrence when they receive conjunctival autograft surgery compared with amniotic membrane transplantation. Thus, such techniques are considered the gold standard surgical procedure for pterygium.

Management of Tenon's capsule remains the subject of debate.[2] The notion that Tenon's capsule gives rise to recurrences has resulted in two approaches, both utilizing wide excision of the pterygium and scar tissue if present:

1. Extensive tenonectomy as advocated by Hirst.[12,20] This large, single surgeon, prospective study was associated with a very low recurrence rate of 0.4%.
2. Medial fornix reconstruction to "seal the gap," creating a barrier between Tenon's capsule and the ocular surface.[21]

An important aspect of both of these techniques is the adequate covering of underlying tissue by epithelial or membranous structures. This raises the possibility that the wound healing response is being modulated, in part by epithelialstromal interactions[22] and perhaps, with adequate graft cover; such extensive excisions are not necessary, particularly if the inflammatory response is controlled.[2,23] Thus in a prospective, randomized controlled study of 36 eyes (34 patients) with primary pterygium treated with the bare sclera technique (a surgical "worst case" scenario), use of topical cyclosporine reduced the recurrence rate by ~ 50% in the control group versus 22 to 44% in the cyclosporine group.[24]

Intensive postoperative anti-inflammatory treatment was used in the extensive tenonectomy studies.[12,20]

7.3 First Principles

The history of conjunctival grafts is appropriately linked to skin grafting both in historical and pathophysiological senses. Skin harvesting and transplantation, described approximately 3,000 years ago with the Hindu Tilemaker Caste (Koomá), in which skin grafting was used to reconstruct noses that were amputated as a means of judicial punishment, has had a central role in reconstructive procedures.[25,26] The development of split-thickness skin grafts by Ollier in 1872[27] and Thiersch in 1886[28] utilizing knowledge of cellular proliferation to expedite the healing process (and to minimize scarring) had important implications for pterygium surgeons. Scarring is a consequence of failure of the wound to properly transition from the regenerative phase to a resolving phase with aberrant repair[29,30]—healing by secondary intention. The resultant uncontrolled inflammatory mediator and growth factor production, deficient generation of anti-inflammatory macrophages, or failed communication between macrophages and epithelial cells, endothelial cells, fibroblasts, and stem or tissue progenitor cells contribute to a state of persistent injury, which may result in fibrosis.[31] Fibrosis and chronic inflammation are deleterious to the health of the ocular surface, and tactics to minimize these phenomena are central to successful pterygium surgery.

7.3.1 Epithelial Mesenchymal Transition

Epithelial mesenchymal transition (EMT), a process where epithelial cells take on characteristics of mesenchymal cells, has been described in both acute and fibrotic cutaneous wound healing of human skin[32] as well as in pterygium.[3,33,34,35] Studies have shown pterygium epithelial cells concurrently expressed epithelial and mesenchymal markers and signaling molecules associated with EMT.[33,34] We have speculated that pterygium fibroblasts may have originated from limbal epithelium via EMT under the influences of transforming growth factor-β (TGF-β) and fibroblast growth factor (FGF)-2 or ultraviolet (UV) exposure.[3] Alternatively, it has been hypothesized that pterygium fibroblasts are recruited from myofibroblasts in the periorbital fibroadipose tissue.[35] This may explain in part why extensive tenonectomy appears to be effective.

Thus a graft of skin or conjunctiva has the potential to reduce the risk of scarring and chronic inflammation via several mechanisms, and this was likely evident to pterygium surgeons early, as surgery for pterygium was being developed.

Traditionally, the standard surgical approach to diseased tissue has been excision, often associated with other destructive/adjunctive therapies. This approach has been reflected in the evolution of pterygium surgery, and at first sight, it would appear that it has only been in recent times that a surgically reconstructive approach has resulted in improved outcomes. Given the well-known restrictive effect of the scarring element of advanced pterygium, with consequent effects on ocular rotation and resultant diplopia, it is perhaps surprising that the widespread adoption of conjunctival autografting had not occurred earlier. In his 1920 book, *Tropical Ophthalmology*, Elliot noted that even primary pterygia could tether the eye medially causing significant binocular diplopia.[36] Yet for many years, the bare sclera technique remained standard practice, despite the eventual documentation of unacceptably high recurrence rates. In 1948, D'Ombrain[37] in describing his technique stated, "A recurrent pterygium is a major ophthalmic problem, often necessitating the use of skin or mucous membrane grafts" and for second recurrences, referred to "the free graft method" described by North.[38] He reasoned that, "in such cases, the sub-conjunctival adhesions are of such density and toughness that tissue planes are lost, and there is danger of actually perforating the sclera if dissection or even separation of the pterygium tissues from the sclera is attempted." North[38] described the use of a limbal skin graft as previously described by Hotz[39,40,41] or a mucous membrane graft as described by Gifford.[42,43] In his experience, the mucous membrane graft was inferior to the skin graft as it encroached onto the cornea and became red and vascularized. He also noted that the skin graft could also grow onto the cornea, forming an "ugly pearly white patch," but this could be safely excised after 6 months.

There is, however, an earlier history of graft repair post pterygium surgery. As early as 1876, Klein[44] described the use of free, full thickness mucous membrane grafts in cases of recurrent pterygium excision where it is impossible to leave sufficient bulbar conjunctiva to cover the defect.

Pollet described a similar technique in 1906.[45] According to Forbes et al,[46] this technique was used for recurrent pterygium but subsequently it was applied both in primary and recurrent cases. Such grafts must have been bulky and given what we know appreciate in regard to the cosmetic implications of this disease[2,12,13]; there would have been motivation to develop more refined and alternative techniques.

As noted, split-skin Ollier–Thiersch grafts were soon adopted for pterygium surgery by Hotz in 1892.[39] It appears that Hotz built on earlier work in which conjunctiva for grafting was harvested from rabbit eyes. Hotz described the healing process after pterygium surgery and noted that where granulation tissue develops in large bare areas post excision, cicatrization is inevitable. In order to "fill the gap" and to "keep the conjunctiva away from the cornea," he noted that as compared to mucous membrane grafts, Thiersch grafts "are much easier to handle and to fit, they need no sutures, they grow better and shrink much less.[41] And as to the appearance, they are as smooth as the surrounding conjunctiva, but look paler, more whitish" and that the "color would blend well with the white of the eyeball." These factors remain of importance to this day. Hotz reported on three cases[39] with grafts as large as 10 × 12 mm being used, with apparent success. Hotz had been of the view that "the substitution of epidermal flaps for epithelial tissue [was] a makeshift to be abandoned as soon as we should find a convenient method of obtaining epithelial grafts, for the ideal aim of our plastic work should be to replace mucous membrane by flaps of the same histologic character."[41] He too referred to work by Gifford,[42] who cut very thin labial flaps using a razor blade (as per Thiersch) with the aid of a specially designed clamp,[43] "so thin that only the epithelium and very little of the sub-adjacent tissue is removed." When healed, the flap "is so much like the conjunctiva that its boundaries are hard to trace." This work can be seen as the prelude to the development of cultivated oral mucosal epithelial transplantation (COMET) for severe ocular surface disease.[47,48] Hotz went on to adopt this technique that was eventually used for both primary and recurrent disease. It is of interest that both of these techniques had some longevity—split-skin grafts were still in use in 1977[49] and split-buccal mucous membrane grafts in 1998.[46]

Various, sometimes ingenious, forms of sliding or rotated conjunctival grafts[50] were developed, but it seems that they were attended by unacceptable recurrence rates and are no longer widely used. In 1888, Hobby devised a sliding conjunctival flap of mobilized adjacent superonasal bulbar conjunctiva to cover bare sclera.[51] This technique also enjoyed some longevity.[52] In Hirst's review,[53] the reported recurrence rates were from < 1 to > 5%, with minimal complications apart from flap retraction. However, as with many pterygium studies, none were prospective, were without controls, and had poor population descriptions.[53] The advantage of this technique, however, is that it attempts to retain limbal integrity, which may be advantageous in preventing recurrence. Another technique for recurrent pterygium was described by Elschnig in 1926[54] in which, after resection, a conjunctival bridge from the opposite limbus was then brought across the cornea in a "bucket handle" to cover the defect, again repairing the limbus (even though the actual temporal limbus was now displaced nasally). These various techniques suffered from the fact that there was still a relative shortage of conjunctival tissue, which could either result in restriction of ocular rotations or a "gap" where healing by second intention, EMT, could result in scarring, chronic inflammation, and lead to recurrence.

The era of autologous conjunctival grafting began with the use of free fragments of conjunctiva used by de Gama Pinto, Gomez-Marques, and de Paula Xavier as described by Rosenthal.[45] Interestingly, this is reminiscent of the modern technique of simple limbal epithelial transplantation (SLET) that is used in the treatment of limbal failure.[55,56] This technique, "mini-SLET," has recently been shown to be efficacious in a small series of 10 patients who underwent pterygium excision with limbal-sparing SLET and who had been followed up on for up to 8 months.[56] It is our impression that with our autologous limbal-conjunctival grafting technique (described later in this chapter), supported with postoperative hyperbaric oxygen, the graft seems to expand after the healing phase. This is contrary to the accepted wisdom of graft shrinkage, but is consistent with observations of minimal skin graft shrinkage under ideal conditions.[57]

A landmark paper in the development of both excision techniques and autoconjunctival grafting was published in 1931 by Gómez-Márquez.[58] He described extensive excision from the pterygium head to the caruncle and subsequent covering of the conjunctival wound with a piece of healthy conjunctiva (▶ Fig. 7.1), taken from the bulbar conjunctiva of the other eye. He cited Duverger,[59] (who also used skin and buccal grafts) who used a

similar autograft technique[60] but who referenced da Gama Pinto who harvested conjunctiva from the same eye. This is perhaps the earliest reference to autoconjunctival grafting as we carry out today.

Before a modern understanding of pterygium pathophysiology, which he acknowledges,[58] he intuited that its propensity to persist, grow, and recur once extirpated, suggested a neoplastic, tumor-like condition, but with distinctive growth patterns (centripetal and superficial). He reasoned that an ideal strategy would be to "completely extirpate the whole tumor mass." While this was possible in its corneal aspect, there is no line of demarcation in its conjunctival aspect, particularly at the caruncular base of the pterygium. Limited excision of the pterygium head he saw "as illusory and unsafe as it would be to destroy an army by simply annihilating its guerrillas, the reserves intended to rebuild the front line." He was concerned about "tumor cells that may exist in the limbal conjunctiva" and "germ"-like cells in apparently normal-looking conjunctiva. He states, "It is therefore necessary to remove this and a large part of the seemingly healthy conjunctiva that prolongs it, in order to prevent the recurrence of pterygium. Proceeding thus, we will have great probability of excising all cells endowed with the specific faculty of replicating in the direction of the cornea and the pterygium will not recur." He took this to the extreme by preferentially harvesting conjunctiva from the unaffected eye (where possible). This method is still used in cases where insufficient conjunctiva remains in eye being treated, usually because of multiple previous failed surgeries. Gómez-Márquez successfully used this technique on recurrent pterygia and noted, "the appearance of an eye operated according to this technique is perfect."

These observations bear some semblance to modern day theory. As discussed, large excisions are recommended by some with extensive tenonectomy[12,20] or "walling off" of Tenon's capsule by over sewing.[21] Such procedures are associated with very low recurrence rates and improved, if not "perfect" cosmesis. The notion of invasive "altered" limbal basal cells has also been confirmed.[61,62,63,64] In excising pterygia, we routinely take ~ 0.5 to 1.00 mm of extra tissue at the limbus in an attempt to clear the limbus of these cells. We have previously postulated[5,65,66] that limbal cells are damaged by peripheral focusing of light being the cornea to the distal limbus, and it is possible that a good part of the limbal circumference is affected. This might account for the types of

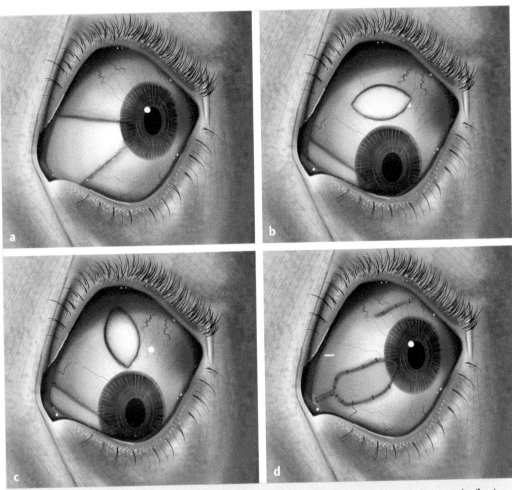

Fig. 7.1 Gómez-Márquez surgical technique, 1931.[58] (a) Extensive excision of the pterygium to the caruncle. (b, c) Conjunctival graft sites from the superior bulbar conjunctiva. Long-axis alignment was determined by extent of conjunctival laxity. (d) Conjunctival graft sutured into position.

recurrences in which tissue invades the cornea above and below the graft (▶ Fig. 7.2). This view is also consistent with the not uncommon finding of dysplastic cells in pterygium specimens.[14,15]

Gómez-Márquez acknowledged some drawbacks of his technique—patient reluctance to have surgery on the unaffected eye and the need to occlude both eyes. He also noted the technical difficulty of the flap rolling up on itself—now soluble by the use of Trypan blue that preferentially stains the stromal aspect of the graft.[2] For these reasons, he confined the technique to recurrent cases.

By 1947, Tagle described a technique in which the excision defect was "covered by a graft obtained from the conjunctival tissue along the superior limbus and anchored with suitable sutures.[67] The donor area is closed with a running stitch." Almost certainly, more widespread usage of this technique occurred with further studies by Barraquer[68] and subsequently,[69] as an understanding of the importance of the limbus and corneal epithelial stem cell biology grew,[70,71,72] and LCAGs evolved (see following text).

Popularization of the CAG technique in North America came with work by Kenyon et al in the 1980s[73] who demonstrated very low recurrence rates in patients with primary or recurrent pterygium. He also described LCAGs, but these were used for other causes of limbal failure.[74] One reason for this may have been concern about inducing limbal failure at the donor site, and since results with conjunctival grafting can be

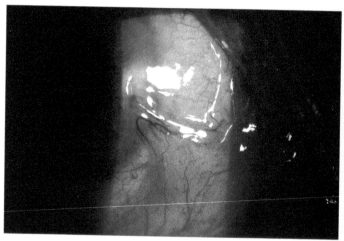

Fig. 7.2 Pterygium recurrence. A tongue of recurrent pterygium invading the cornea inferior to the lower border of a conjunctival graft. This type of recurrence could be due to inadequate excision of diseased limbal tissue above or below where the pterygium body crosses the limbus. It has been hypothesized that altered/diseased limbal stem cells could reside in these locations and give rise to this aspect of the recurrence. (Image courtesy of Dr Laurence Sullivan.)

excellent, limbal-conjunctival grafting has not been widely adopted. However, the long-standing concept that corneal epithelial stem cells reside mainly in the limbus has been challenged[75,76]; it has been shown that basal cells of bulbar conjunctival epithelium share a similar expression pattern of stem cell–associated markers to the limbal epithelium.[77] This may help explain the success of CAGs and why a limbal area appears to reform when conjunctival grafts are used and that there are apparently few cases of limbal failure at the donor site when LCAGs have been used.

The LCAG technique has evolved, and in general, its use is associated with very low recurrence rates with few reports of complications.[18,78,79,80,81,82] Many authors use this procedure for recurrent pterygium, and in one randomized, prospective, parallel-group clinical trial, the recurrence rate for the CAG group was significantly higher at 10.0% versus the LCAG group with a recurrence rate of 1%.[83] In another randomized controlled trial with a decade of follow-up, patients treated with excision, intraoperative 0.02% MMC, and local conjunctival closure had a recurrence rate of 25.5% as compared to the LCAG group with a recurrence rate of 6.9%. Similar data was presented with 12 years follow-up.[84] Post MMC, eyes had more fibrovascular tissue in the conjunctival bed. This study also found that in the LCAG group all of the recurrences took place within 1 year, for the MMC group there was an ongoing recurrence rate beyond the first year.[85] This is consistent with concerns previously raised about MMC (see later in this chapter).

7.3.2 Author's Technique

Anesthesia is usually achieved with a peribulbar block using a long-acting anesthetic. Brimonidine eye drops are applied to act as a vasoconstrictor and have the advantage of not dilating the pupil like adrenaline. Half-strength povidone is applied and careful lash-excluding draping is carried out.

1. The pterygium head is excised using a 23-gauge (G) needle-tip technique[86] (▶ Fig. 7.3a and **Video 7.1**) minimizing the amount of corneal tissue excised. Smoothing is not carried out since this removes more tissue unnecessarily, given that perhaps the best smoothing agent is resurfacing with corneal epithelium. This technique also allows complete removal of pterygium tissue from the cornea; this is of importance since residual tissue left behind can be a cause of concern of patient dissatisfaction. If the surgeon is right-handed, when operating on a left eye, the microscope is moved so that the pterygium head dissection is carried out from the side, following which it is then moved so that the superior bulbar conjunctiva and limbus can be approached from above. Care is taken as the limbus is approached, as given the change in radius of curvature, it is important to avoid damage to the sclera. Instead, the corneal dissection merges into the limbal subconjunctival/sub-pterygium space. The body of the pterygium is then excised, taking care to excise tissue for about 1 mm above and below these sites where the pterygium crosses the limbus as described above.

2. Carrying out an extensive but superficial excision, removing inflamed tissue as far as the

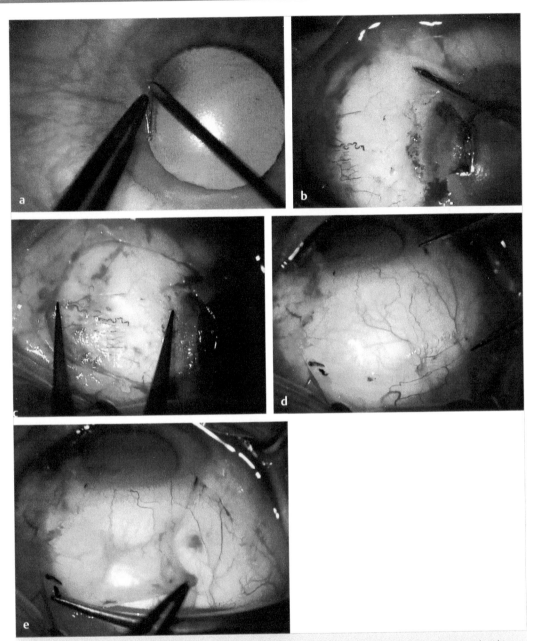

Fig. 7.3 (a) Pterygium head excision using a 23-gauge needle tip. After the leading edge of the pterygium head is delineated, vertical retraction reveals the point of attachment of the pterygium to the cornea. Touching this junction with the needle tip causes a "splitting" in a plane that is neither too superficial nor too deep. (b) Bleeding is controlled by using an intraocular diathermy tip, to minimize collateral tissue and particularly, vascular damage. (c) Excision defect size is measured with calipers—the horizontal extent is measured with the eye in forced abduction. (d) A typically trapezoidal conjunctival graft is marked out at the superior limbus and on the bulbar conjunctiva, reflecting the size and shape of the excision defect and oversizing by ~ 0.5 mm in length and breadth. (e) A thin conjunctival graft is dissected with spring scissors. (*continued*)

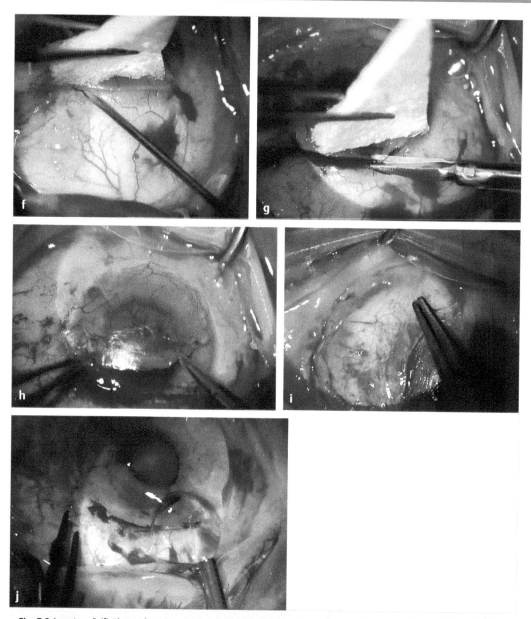

Fig. 7.3 (*continued*) (**f**) The graft is then folded down over the cornea, still hinged at the limbus, and the short end of a stroll wedge is used to retract the graft inferiorly so that there is some tension at the limbal hinge. The limbus is dissected to ~ 50% of the vertical extent of the palisades of Vogt using a 23-gauge needle tip. (**g**) The limbal-conjunctival graft is amputated at the "split" limbus using Vannas scissors. (**h**) The graft is picked up at the limbal edges with non-toothed tying forceps. The epithelial surface is in contact with the corneal surface, and the graft is slid across to the site of pterygium excision defect and inverted so that the epithelial aspect is superficial. (**i**) The graft limbal edge is aligned with the limbal aspect of the defect and secured into position. Absorbable 10–0 polyglycolic acid (PolySyn GA-966, Sharpoint) sutures are preferred. Small bites of episclera/sclera are taken at the limbus, and all knots are buried. (**j**) An extended wear balafilcon A contact lens (PureVision, Bausch and Lomb) is placed at the end of the procedure.

plica, if it is still present and if not, just short of the caruncle. Check ligaments and the medial rectus muscle capsule are avoided in primary pterygium. Excess Tenon's capsule underlying this excision area is also trimmed, but "Tenon's fishing" by pulling on exposed connective tissue is avoided.

Bleeding is controlled with judicious use of an intraocular diathermy (▶ Fig. 7.3b)—particular care is taken to check for bleeding along and under the cut edges of the conjunctiva, especially in the region of the caruncle. Subgraft hemorrhages, while uncommon, have originated form this area.

3. The size of excised area is measured with calipers (▶ Fig. 7.3c) and its horizontal extent is estimated with the eye in forced abduction and graft size marked (▶ Fig. 7.3d) on the superior bulbar conjunctiva. Graft dissection to the superior limbus is not infrequent, and an assistant can be helpful.

4. A thin flap is cut with Westcott-style spring scissors (Martin [35–822–11]) (Fig. M5) (▶ Fig. 7.3e) and oversized by ~ 0.5 mm. The dissected graft is then folded down over the cornea, and if necessary, excess Tenon's capsule can be trimmed from this exposed graft under surface. A stroll wedge (short end) is used to retract the graft inferiorly, and the limbus is further dissected using the tip of a fresh 23-G needle (▶ Fig. 7.3f). Perforating vessels in this area can result in bleeding, controlled with a second wedge. The aim with this maneuver is to split the limbus, leaving behind sufficient palisadal tissue and stem cells to obviate deficiency. The graft is then detached from the limbus (▶ Fig. 7.3g) with Vannas scissors, taking care to include tissue with a crenellated appearance, an indication that tissue is from the palisades of Vogt. The graft is then glided across a balanced salt-lubricated cornea, using non-toothed tying forceps (▶ Fig. 7.3h), flipped over and placed in the wound created by the pterygium excision (▶ Fig. 7.3i). As indicated, if graft orientation is lost, Trypan blue can be used to check. The graft is sutured in place commencing with limbal sutures, and this, I preferred to glue, given the large size of these grafts.

5. To reduce postoperative pain and to protect the limbus, an extended-wear contact lens is placed at the end of the procedure (▶ Fig. 7.3j). Lenses made of balafilcon A are used since these lenses do not do well supporting the cell growth that occurs in the week that the lens is left in situ,[87] and this is likely to be less "sticky" to the ocular surface. We have also commenced the use of cyclopentolate 1% eye drops at the end of the case, in an attempt to further reduce postoperative pain.[88] Interestingly, in an earlier era, atropine was used for this purpose.[37]

6. Postoperatively, chloramphenicol, Prednefrin forte, and preservative-free diclofenac eye drops are used four times daily and usually tapered after 1 week, with treatment lasting typically 4 to 6 weeks. Topical treatment is prolonged if excessive inflammation occurs, and topical cyclosporine may also be introduced or restarted if the patient was being treated for dry eye syndrome preoperatively. This treatment regime has been used since a key factor in recurrence is postoperative inflammation (see below), and this treatment regime aims to keep this at a minimum. Patients need to be watched carefully since nonsteroidal anti-inflammatory drugs (NSAIDs) can induce corneal melting, and this seems to occur at the junction of the graft with the limbus. At the first sign of an epithelial defect, topical NSAID treatment is ceased, steroid treatment is further reduced, and lubrication is increased. If the graft edge is raised, an extended-wear contact lens is placed.

In recurrent pterygium cases, forced duction assists in determining the extent of tissue fibrosis between the recurrence site and medial rectus muscle and surrounding tissue. In such cases, the medial rectus muscle is isolated and appropriate dissection with excision of Tenon's capsule carried out. Forced duction is repeated to make sure that all fibrotic bands are cut. In such cases, extensive grafts are required, and if there is insufficient bulbar conjunctiva in the eye undergoing pterygium excision, donor tissue can be taken from the other eye. This can be anticipated preoperatively and discussed with the patient prior to surgery. All such cases receive hyperbaric oxygen for a week after surgery.[89]

By splitting the limbus, we have aimed to avoid issues with localized stem cell failure, deficient epithelial healing,[90,91] and Mooren's ulcer[92] that have been reported at graft harvest sites. To date, we have not encountered these complications with our technique.

7.3.3 Inflammation

Inflammation is central to pterygium surgical response and pathogenesis, as well as the extent of signs, symptoms, growth, and recurrence.[2] Inadequate use of postoperative topical steroids was associated with almost tripling of the recurrence rate.[23] In Hirst's studies[12,20] for which very low recurrence rates were reported, topical steroids were used every 2 hours for the first 3 weeks with treatment extended to 9 weeks. As discussed, postoperative topical cyclosporine has been shown to halve the recurrence rate while using the high-recurrence rate bare sclera technique.[24] It remains to be seen whether cyclosporine is as effective in the more sophisticated surgical techniques, but it has a safer side effect profile.

We have found that a risk factor for recurrence is dry eye syndrome and assess all of our pterygium patients for this condition.[93] If surgery is planned, the dry eye syndrome is treated aggressively, prior to surgery. Following pterygium surgery, both symptoms and signs of dry eye often recede, as has previously been reported.[11]

7.3.4 Antimetabolites

Antimetabolites are not used since this technique has a recurrence rate of < 1% (practice audit) and is consistent with reports where a similar technique has been utilized.[18,80,81,82,83] It also avoids the potential and sometimes substantial risks posed by such treatments both in the short term but also particularly in the longer term.[2,94] One view is that the long-term complications of pterygium surgery that involved destructive procedures, such as use of beta irradiation or MMC, relate to failure of tissue maintenance. As noted, there appears to be more fibrovascular tissue at the surgical site and recurrences beyond 1 year where MMC has been used,[12] which may be significant given that there is a 97% chance that a recurrence will occur within 12 months.[95] Scleral plaques (often colonized by microorganisms), deficiency/necrosis[96,97,98] have been associated with severe infections, including fungal and pseudomonas infections with significant morbidity. By resurfacing the eye with healthy conjunctiva/limbal-conjunctiva with regenerative capacity,[1] part of the aim is to ensure long-term globe integrity, thereby avoiding such complications.

7.3.5 Novel Observations

Adjunctive Use of Hyperbaric Oxygen

Some insight into graft vascularization, a key to graft success, can be derived from considering the graft bed and the consequences of previous surgery. In 2011, we reported on conjunctival autograft failure in cases treated for recurrent pterygium with either beta radiation or MMC.[99] Since irradiation can result in an obliterative endarteritis in exposed tissues, it is commonly recognized as a factor in graft failure elsewhere. The aim of using irradiation in the management of pterygium is to destroy episcleral vessels that could potentially provide nutrition for a recurrent pterygium.[100] Furthermore, there may be similarities between irradiation and antimetabolites—MMC is cytotoxic to vascular endothelial cells in vitro[101] and is seen as being "radiomimetic."[2] Reasoning that these adjunctive treatments along with surgery induced scarring had damaged the vascular bed from which a graft would be revascularized, and also since it has been shown that following CAG, the graft is perfused from the underlying episcleral vascular bed as early as 1 week postoperatively,[102] we proposed the use of adjuvant hyperbaric oxygen therapy in such cases.[89] Hyperbaric oxygen has been used to support "at-risk" grafts and flaps with success for this purpose in other anatomical sites,[103,104] and we have previously reviewed mechanisms of action.[89] In our study of 39 eyes with recurrent pterygium, 18 had a known history of exposure to beta radiation or MMC, and within a mean follow-up of 23.1 months, there was a single recurrence. For the remaining 21 eyes, there were no recurrences within a mean follow-up of 19.4 months. There were no significant complications associated with the hyperbaric treatment. We concluded that since in general terms, there are increased recurrence rates for the removal of already recurrent pterygia,[53] adjuvant hyperbaric oxygen treatment should be considered in the surgical management of recurrent pterygium.

Effects of Concurrent Treatment with Vascular Endothelial Growth Factor Inhibitors

Further insight into LCAG/CAG vascularization can be derived from our report of a patient who underwent pterygium with an LCAG and developed graft dehiscence with melting of the graft and underlying sclera at approximately 2 weeks post-surgery.[105] The patient was receiving intravitreal anti-vascular endothelial growth factor (VEGF) injections and underwent pterygium surgery prior to undergoing cataract surgery. This was necessitated by the fact that cataract had reduced both vision and visualization of the retina. Since pterygium, cataract, and macular degeneration are all age-related and, arguably, UV light exposure-related diseases, these conditions can coexist and may all require treatment in an individual patient.

It transpires that VEGF inhibitors, while generally well tolerated, can be associated with wound healing issues, both in ocular and non-ocular tissue.[105] This occurs not just via inhibition of vascularization but also inhibition of cell–cell adhesion, effect on endothelial cells and platelets and an angio-fibrotic switch mechanism.[106] Of interest is that local application VEGF may improve graft survival,[107] and this intervention could be considered in LCAG/CAG in the future.

Timing of surgery following anti-VEGF injections requires consideration—bevacizumab has an average half-life of 20 days (range 11–50 days), and residual drug exposure can persist for weeks to months. After intravitreal injections, subconjunctival reflux can occur in ~ 30% of cases, and there is a mean drug residence time ~ 10 to 13 days. While the optimal interval from interruption of anti-angiogenesis treatment to surgery has not been determined, most clinical trials with anti-angiogenesis therapies require at least 28 days from any major surgery before starting treatment. While a 60-day delay is safer, this is likely to be impractical in most settings.[105]

Graft-site Healing

While it is possible to create very thin LCAGs with this method, it is impossible to not breach Tenon's capsule, which is adherent to the conjunctiva in a "Velcro-like" fashion. While healing of the graft donor site is usually satisfactory, occasionally, scarring occurs, and this can affect ocular motility with consequent diplopia[108] (▶ Fig. 7.4). Milder forms of inflammation can be seen without significant scarring (▶ Fig. 7.5). Largely to reduce pain and discomfort, attempts have been made to also cover the bare area of graft donor site by direct suturing,[58] amniotic membrane,[109] and polyethylene glycol hydrogel,[110] with varying degrees of success. It is of interest that this area usually heals rapidly, and at least in the initial phase, cells grow from the limbus to meet the superior aspect of the graft site. The appearance is that of corneal epithelium (▶ Fig. 7.6), perhaps accounting for the rapid healing rate. Typically, in our experience, a second graft re-harvested from this site is not always possible or difficult due to scarring (▶ Fig. 7.4), although it has been described.[12] Despite the fact that this area can have a relatively normal appearance, invariably the conjunctiva is adherent to underlying layers and a second procedure runs the risk of further scarring. Scarring at this site also limits options for glaucoma drainage surgery should this be required in the future, although with the advent of minimally invasive glaucoma devices,[111] this may become less problematic.

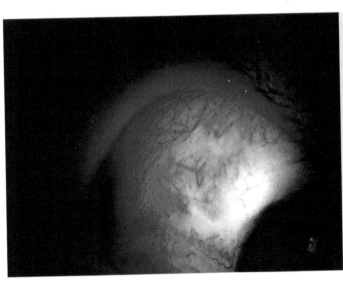

Fig. 7.4 Inflammation and early scarring affecting the superotemporal bulbar conjunctiva following a re-harvesting of limbal-conjunctival autografting (LCAG) for a recurrent pterygium. This caused horizontal diplopia in extremes of horizontal gaze.

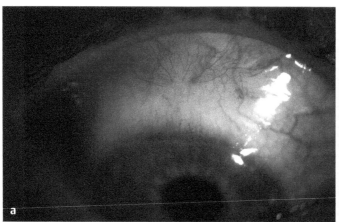

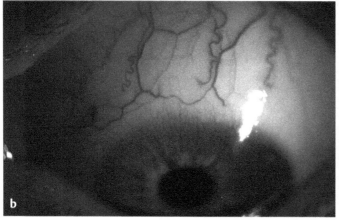

Fig. 7.5 (a) Healed superior bulbar region following limbal-conjunctival autografting (LCAG) in a right eye. Note that the superior area of conjunctiva appears somewhat inflamed, and the area just superior to the limbus appears less inflamed (see ▶ Fig. 7.6). The limbus shows evidence of where the limbal aspect of the graft was harvested, with evidence of some residual limbus left in situ. (a) The left, unoperated fellow eye to that shown in (b). The superior bulbar region and limbus are of normal appearance in contrast to the corresponding areas in (a). LCAG, limbal-conjunctival autografting.

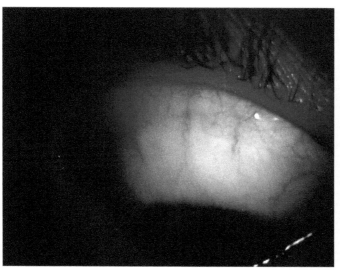

Fig. 7.6 Healed limbal-conjunctival autografting (LCAG) donor site. Note the relatively avascular superior paralimbal tissue, which has grown out from the limbus. This area has the clinical appearance of corneal epithelium. This phenomenon is also evident in **7.5a**.

In light of these observations, we sought an improved technique for creating CAG and LCAGs that would minimize the risk of scarring and that would more precisely size the graft than current methods. To do this, we first developed an in vitro porcine eye model, which was also developed in order to train novice surgeons. We then went on to develop a femtosecond laser-based technique to create such grafts.

7.3.6 Complications Relating to LCAG/CAG Surgery

This case is instructive in how to deal with a significant complication of this surgery. The patient was commenced on hyperbaric oxygen treatment for 21 days, and topical doxycycline, chloramphenicol, steroids and unpreserved lubricants were continued. No further anti-VEGF injections were given during this time and the macula continued to be observed and was stable. The scleral melt slowly resolved and the ocular surface re-epithelialized.[105] We would take a similar approach with managing surgically induced necrotizing scleritis (SINS) for which systemic immunosuppression has recently been proposed.[112] This approach, however, could be problematic since there is a recent report of a case of *Purpureocillium lilacinum* endophthalmitis in a case of post pterygium SINS, treated with infliximab.[113]

As discussed, unsuspected neoplasia is present not uncommonly in pterygium surgical specimens,[14,15] and we believe that all pterygia specimens should be submitted for histopathologic examination. It is possible that with larger excision specimens, such changes will be detected and more completely excised. If neoplasia is detected, more frequent postoperative surveillance is recommended; however, such cases can be treated with topical interferon with or without retinoic acid, a very effective medical treatment for OSSN.[114] We have managed a case in which, despite a suspicious pathology (reported as "consistent with pterygium showing focal low-grade dysplasia"), this was not followed up[8] when 2 years later the patient noted a whitening of the nasal aspect of his cornea. The patient presented 4 years later with mucoepidermoid (adenosquamous) SCC disease involving the limbus and cornea with intraocular extension. The eye was enucleated, confirming the diagnosis and demonstrating clear surgical margins. There was no local recurrence or metastasis after 7 years of follow up.

The possibility of limbal failure and the development of Mooren's ulcer at the graft donor site have been discussed.[92]

Granulomas can develop either at graft or donor sites but are relatively uncommon. While they can be simply excised, recently, treatment with topical beta-blockers has been reported.[115] Proposed mechanisms of action include vasoconstriction, inhibition of angiogenesis, and the induction of apoptosis in proliferating endothelial cells.

7.3.7 Training of Surgeons in Graft Techniques

Since the LCAG/CAG technique is associated with excellent outcomes—relatively low recurrence rates, excellent cosmesis, and minor complications—it is important that there is adequate training of novice surgeons in this technique, particularly since in various parts of the world, pterygium prevalence is high. The technique is time consuming and technically difficult, and this may be reflected in the fact that there are significantly higher recurrence rates in trainee and less experienced surgeons.[10] We saw a need for and went on to develop a cadaveric porcine eye model for both teaching the surgical technique of CAG/LCAG creation as well as for acquiring suturing skills.[116] We found that 24-week-old pig eyes are subjectively similar to that of a young human eye. Our aim was also to use this model to develop improved graft techniques.

We were able to demonstrate that a medical student could be taught this technique and that graft thickness be reduced significantly with experience so that after approximately 60 grafts, a graft thickness of 87 ± 23 μm could be achieved. The thickness of human bulbar conjunctiva epithelium has been found to be 47.3 ± 8.4 μm (standard deviation [SD]) with a stromal thickness of 190.8 ± 47.5 μm, using optical coherence tomography,[117] so that these graft thicknesses represent a good result, with minimal Tenon's incursion. The median time of graft creation also fell from more than 3 minutes for the first 10 grafts to 2 minutes for the last 10 grafts.

7.3.8 Femtosecond Laser-Assisted Conjunctival Flaps

Femtosecond lasers have been utilized in ophthalmology for almost 2 decades, initially in corneal refractive surgery and more recently in cataract surgery.[118,119,120] In refractive surgery, they are superior to mechanical microkeratomes, rapidly allowing creation of corneal flaps of precise diameter, thickness, and uniformity.[121,122] It seemed that these characteristics were precisely what were required in CAG/LCAG creation even though we were dealing with conjunctiva, a vascularized, translucent tissue of different consistency and transparency to the cornea, for which these lasers were originally designed. We evaluated the feasibility of using this technology to create ideal, Tenon's free grafts and furthermore to evaluate teaching aspects of this procedure.[123,124,125]

Initially, we utilized our cadaveric porcine eye model[116,123] and the Ziemer LDV Z8 (Ziemer Ophthalmic Systems AG, Port, Switzerland), a low energy (50–2500 nJ) high frequency (0.1–10 MHz) femtosecond laser, with a large numerical aperture that enables it to cut through translucent tissue such as the conjunctiva.[123] Such lasers also minimize cell loss and inflammation, of potential concern in creating CAG/LCAGs.[126] We were able to show that flaps cut at 60 μm were consistently closer to the intended thickness than those cut at 100 μm. The performance of an experienced versus an inexperienced surgeon was compared, and we

were able to show that they produced flaps of comparable thickness and variability. No buttonholes or tags occurred during surgery. The mean time to create 60-μm flaps was 18.1 ± 2.2 seconds. This study also demonstrated maintenance of conjunctival stromal vasculature in these thin grafts with small- and medium-sized stromal blood vessels being demonstrated with immunohistochemistry. This is of importance since in free skin grafts, these vessels are "reutilized" and are associated with early vascularization and graft survival.[127] Thus, the consideration of very thin conjunctival grafts should take inclusion of this vasculature into account.

Having optimized laser parameters and techniques in our porcine model, we went on to commence a clinical trial to evaluate the feasibility and safety for FLAPS in humans (NCT02866968) that was approved by the SingHealth Centralised Institutional Review Board (R1361/47/2016). In this study, we treated six eyes of five patients with FLAPS[124] with early promising results (▶ Fig. 7.7, ▶ Fig. 7.8, ▶ Fig. 7.9, ▶ Fig. 7.10). The technique has been described in detail; however, after pterygium excision, the defect was measured with a caliper and the Z8 programmed to dissect a corresponding

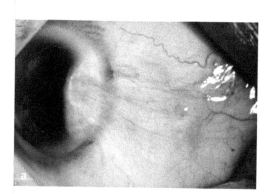

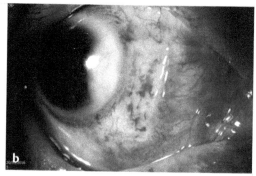

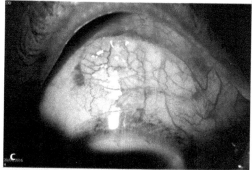

Fig. 7.7 (a) Preop and (b,c) postop photos at day 1 of a patient who underwent femtosecond laser-assisted conjunctival flaps (FLAPS).

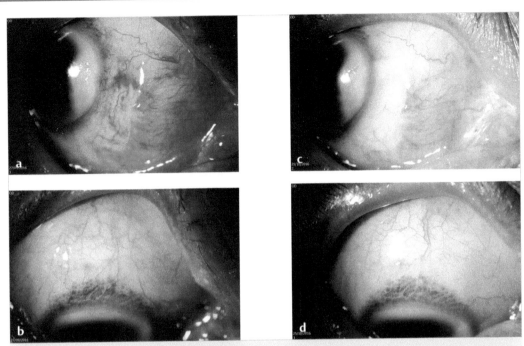

Fig. 7.8 The same patient showing the conjunctival autografting (CAG) site and donor sites at **(a,b)** 1 week and **(c,d)** 1 month. There is minimal inflammation at the CAG donor site, even at 1 week.

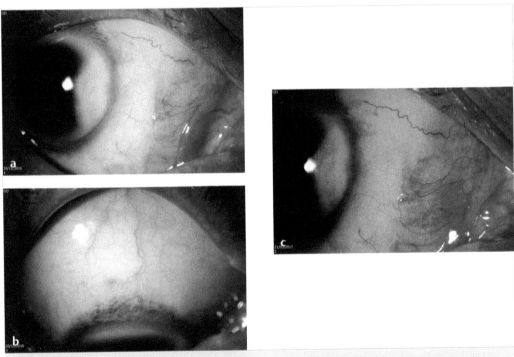

Fig. 7.9 Corresponding images at **(a,b)** 3 and **(c)** 6 months. There is no sign of inflammation or scarring at the conjunctival autografting (CAG) door site at 3 months. The graft has healed with no sign of inflammation.

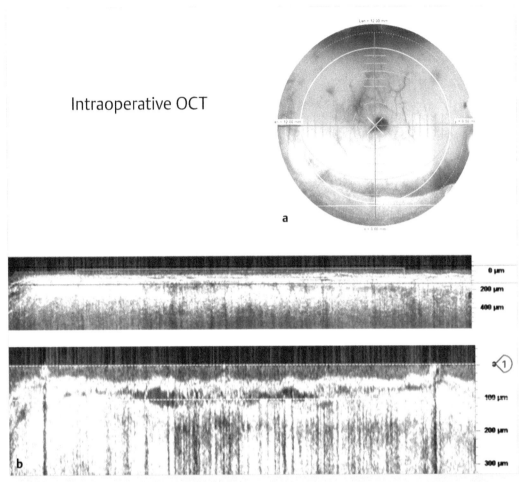

Fig. 7.10 (**a**) Shows applanation of the laser head onto the ocular surface. The conjunctiva is marked to enable centration with the laser head. (**b**) shows the intraoperative optical coherence tomography (OCT) on the Z8 laser, before (upper) and after (lower) cutting of the conjunctiva. The resection plane can be seen in the lower scan as a dark area at approximately 65 μm from the surface.

ellipsoid of superior bulbar conjunctiva. After positioning and laser centration, the ocular surface was gently applanated with the laser head, and no suction was required. Completeness of graft dissection was confirmed by intraoperative optical coherence tomography (OCT) (▶ Fig. 7.10). The CAG was then lifted from its bed with forceps and was placed stromal-side-up on the cornea, and graft thickness was measured by OCT. Fibrin glue was then applied to the graft and the scleral bed, and the CAG was inverted and positioned into the surgical defect. Graft sizes varied from 6 × 8 mm to 7 × 10 mm, and no buttonholes or CAG tags occurred during surgery. The mean laser dissection time was 19.5 ±1.2 (17–20) seconds, and the

time to remove the laser-prepared CAG from the conjunctival stromal bed and to unfold it onto the cornea was 10.3 ± 3.8 (5–15) seconds—a substantial saving in time as compared to conventional surgery. The graft material is so thin that gluing is the preferred method of attachment, since sutures could damage the graft edges.

We reported a mean follow-up of 35.8 ± 38.0 (8–106) days, and the epithelium healed at the graft donor site within 1 week in all patients (▶ Fig. 7.8). In this follow-up period, no postoperative complication or recurrences occurred, but it is acknowledged that longer follow-up will be needed in the evaluation of this technique. There was no evidence of scarring at the conjunctival graft harvest site, allowing the real possibility of re-harvesting and no impediment to glaucoma drainage surgery if required in the future. This technique offers the advantages of ultrathin, uniform CAGs, with minimal (if any) breach of Tenon's capsule that are reproducible, consistent, and relatively independent of prior experience with either pterygium or laser surgery. Future development of purpose-designed ocular surface modules may also allow larger grafts that also allow inclusion of limbal tissue and the possibility of custom-sizing after acute measurement of the pterygium resection site. This technique has the potential to further standardize the procedure as has occurred with cataract surgery and which may be occurring with minimally invasive glaucoma procedures, to lift success rates across a range of surgeon abilities.

7.4 Conclusion

Pterygium surgery has evolved from initially destructive to reconstructive procedures, since destructive procedures were and are accompanied by high recurrence rates and suboptimal outcomes. The development of the CAG/LCAG technique, with the aim of minimizing inflammation and scarring in an attempt to rehabilitate the ocular surface to a more normal state, has been central to the success of this surgery. Such techniques have developed over the last 125 years from split-skin and mucous membrane grafts to sophisticated, femtosecond laser-fashioned grafts of precise size and thickness. With modern anti-inflammatory treatment regimes, as well as adjunctive use of hyperbaric oxygen in high-risk cases, graft survival with minimal scarring is the norm. Such less invasive procedures help us complete our mission of restoring ocular surface anatomy, function, and cosmesis and in so doing, alleviate all associated symptoms, painlessly. Treating early will also reduce the risk of astigmatism. While the use of femtosecond lasers in pterygium surgery will be debated, one should not lose sight of the fact that in the past, pterygium surgery has been trivialized, at some considerable cost to our patients. The very rapid and accurate creation of CAG/LCAGs made possible by this technology is attended by rapid recovery and minimal scarring. We believe that this represents a significant advance. If adopted more widely, equipment costs are likely to fall, and taking into account the savings in operating room time, we may also be able to carry out this surgery cost effectively.

References

[1] Coroneo MT. Paradigm shifts, peregrinations and pixies in ophthalmology: Ida Mann lecture 2015. Clin Exp Ophthalmol. 2018; 46(3):280–297

[2] Coroneo MT, Chui JJY. Pterygium. In: Holland EJ, Mannis MJ, W. Lee WB, eds. Ocular Surface Disease: Cornea, Conjunctiva and Tear Film. London: Elsevier Saunders; 2013:125–144

[3] Chui J, Di Girolamo N, Wakefield D, Coroneo MT. The pathogenesis of pterygium: current concepts and their therapeutic implications. Ocul Surf. 2008; 6(1):24–43

[4] Chui J, Coroneo MT. Pterygium pathogenesis, actinic damage, and recurrence. In: Hovanesian J, ed. Pterygium: Techniques and Technologies for Surgical Success. Thorofare NJ: Slack; 2011

[5] Coroneo M. Ultraviolet radiation and the anterior eye. Eye Contact Lens. 2011; 37(4):214–224

[6] Villegas EA, Alcón E, Artal P. Minimum amount of astigmatism that should be corrected. J Cataract Refract Surg. 2014; 40(1):13–19

[7] Cao X-G, Li X-X, Bao Y-Z. Relationship between pterygium and age-related cataract among rural populations living in two different latitude areas in China. Int J Clin Exp Med. 2017; 10(2):3494–3501

[8] Mendoza PR, Craven CM, Ip MH, et al. Conjunctival squamous cell carcinoma with corneal stromal invasion in presumed pterygia: a case series. Ocul Oncol Pathol. 2018; 4(4): 240–249

[9] Seregard S, Kock E. Squamous spindle cell carcinoma of the conjunctiva. Fatal outcome of a pterygium-like lesion. Acta Ophthalmol Scand. 1995; 73(5):464–466

[10] Ti SE, Chee SP, Dear KB, Tan DT. Analysis of variation in success rates in conjunctival autografting for primary and recurrent pterygium. Br J Ophthalmol. 2000; 84(4):385–389

[11] Li M, Zhang M, Lin Y, et al. Tear function and goblet cell density after pterygium excision. Eye (Lond). 2007; 21(2):224–228

[12] Hirst LW. Recurrent pterygium surgery using pterygium extended removal followed by extended conjunctival transplant: recurrence rate and cosmesis. Ophthalmology. 2009; 116(7):1278–1286

[13] Hirst LW. Cosmesis after pterygium extended removal followed by extended conjunctival transplant as assessed by a new, web-based grading system. Ophthalmology. 2011; 118 (9):1739–1746

[14] Chui J, Coroneo MT, Tat LT, Crouch R, Wakefield D, Di Girolamo N. Ophthalmic pterygium: a stem cell disorder with premalignant features. Am J Pathol. 2011; 178(2):817–827

[15] Hirst LW, Axelsen RA, Schwab I. Pterygium and associated ocular surface squamous neoplasia. Arch Ophthalmol. 2009; 127(1):31–32

[16] Perra MT, Colombari R, Maxia C, et al. Finding of conjunctival melanocytic pigmented lesions within pterygium. Histopathology. 2006; 48(4):387–393

[17] Kaufman SC, Jacobs DS, Lee WB, Deng SX, Rosenblatt MI, Shtein RM. Options and adjuvants in surgery for pterygium: a report by the American Academy of Ophthalmology. Ophthalmology. 2013; 120(1):201–208

[18] Masters JS, Harris DJ , Jr. Low recurrence rate of pterygium after excision with conjunctival limbal autograft: a retrospective study with long-term follow-up. Cornea. 2015; 34 (12):1569–1572

[19] Clearfield E, Muthappan V, Wang X, Kuo IC. Conjunctival autograft for pterygium. Cochrane Database Syst Rev. 2016; 2:CD011349

[20] Hirst LW. Prospective study of primary pterygium surgery using pterygium extended removal followed by extended conjunctival transplantation. Ophthalmology. 2008; 115 (10):1663–1672

[21] Liu J, Fu Y, Xu Y, Tseng SC. New grading system to improve the surgical outcome of multirecurrent pterygia. Arch Ophthalmol. 2012; 130(1):39–49

[22] Notara M, Shortt AJ, Galatowicz G, Calder V, Daniels JT. IL6 and the human limbal stem cell niche: a mediator of epithelial-stromal interaction. Stem Cell Res (Amst). 2010; 5(3): 188–200

[23] Yaisawang S, Piyapattanakorn P. Role of post-operative topical corticosteroids in recurrence rate after pterygium excision with conjunctival autograft. J Med Assoc Thai. 2003; 86 Suppl 2:S215–S223

[24] Turan-Vural E, Torun-Acar B, Kivanc SA, Acar S. The effect of topical 0.05% cyclosporine on recurrence following pterygium surgery. Clin Ophthalmol. 2011; 5:881–885

[25] Hauben DJ, Baruchin A, Mahler A. On the history of the free skin graft. Ann Plast Surg. 1982; 9(3):242–245

[26] Davis JS. The story of plastic surgery. Ann Surg. 1941; 113 (5):641–656

[27] Ollier L X E L. Greffes cutanées ou autoplastiques. Bulletin de l'Académie de médecine, Paris,. 1872; 2(sér 1):243–250

[28] Klasen HJ. History of free skin grafting. Knowledge of Empiricism? Berlin, New York: Springer-Verlag; 1891

[29] Yates CC, Hebda P, Wells A. Skin wound healing and scarring: fetal wounds and regenerative restitution. Birth Defects Res C Embryo Today. 2012; 96(4):325–333

[30] Harty M, Neff AW, King MW, Mescher AL. Regeneration or scarring: an immunologic perspective. Dev Dyn. 2003; 226 (2):268–279

[31] Wynn TA, Vannella KM. Macrophages in tissue repair, regeneration, and fibrosis. Immunity. 2016; 44(3):450–462

[32] Yan C, Grimm WA, Garner WL, et al. Epithelial to mesenchymal transition in human skin wound healing is induced by tumor necrosis factor-alpha through bone morphogenic protein-2. Am J Pathol. 2010; 176(5):2247–2258

[33] Kato N, Shimmura S, Kawakita T, et al. Beta-catenin activation and epithelial-mesenchymal transition in the pathogenesis of pterygium. Invest Ophthalmol Vis Sci. 2007; 48 (4):1511–1517

[34] Kase S, Osaki M, Sato I, et al. Immunolocalisation of E-cadherin and beta-catenin in human pterygium. Br J Ophthalmol. 2007; 91(9):1209–1212

[35] Touhami A, Di Pascuale MA, Kawatika T, et al. Characterisation of myofibroblasts in fibrovascular tissues of primary and recurrent pterygia. Br J Ophthalmol. 2005; 89(3):269–274

[36] Elliot RH. Tropical Ophthalmology. London: Hentry Frowde Hodder & Stoughton; 1920

[37] D'Ombrain A. The surgical treatment of pterygium. Br J Ophthalmol. 1948; 32(2):65–71

[38] North AL. The treatment of pterygium. Trans Ophthalmol Soc Aust. 1940; 2:81–83

[39] Hotz FC. A few experiments with Thiersch's grafts in the operation for pterygium. JAMA. 1892; 19(11):297–298

[40] Hotz FC. Ueber die Verwendung Thiersch'scher Hautlappchen bei der Pterygium-Operation. Klin Monatsbl Augenheilkd. 1897; 35:175–177

[41] Hotz FC. On the use of epithelial grafts for replacing the ocular conjunctiva. JAMA. 1898; 31(14):775–777

[42] Gifford H. On the Use of Epithelial Lip-flaps and Half Skin-flaps in Eye Surgery. Ophthalmic Res. 1897; 6:640–642

[43] Gifford H. The treatment of recurrent pterygium. Ophthalmic Res. 1909; 28:1–8

[44] Klein: Zur Operation des Pterygium und zur Transplantation von Scheimhaut. Allgem Weiner Med Zeitung. 1876:3–4

[45] Rosenthal JW. Chronology of pterygium therapy. Am J Ophthalmol. 1953; 36(11):1601–1616

[46] Forbes J, Collin R, Dart J. Split thickness buccal mucous membrane grafts and beta irradiation in the treatment of recurrent pterygium. Br J Ophthalmol. 1998; 82(12):1420–1423

[47] Nakamura T, Inatomi T, Sotozono C, Amemiya T, Kanamura N, Kinoshita S. Transplantation of cultivated autologous oral mucosal epithelial cells in patients with severe ocular surface disorders. Br J Ophthalmol. 2004; 88(10):1280–1284

[48] Prabhasawat P, Ekpo P, Uiprasertkul M, et al. Long-term result of autologous cultivated oral mucosal epithelial transplantation for severe ocular surface disease. Cell Tissue Bank. 2016; 17(3):491–503

[49] Wong WW. Behavior of skin grafts in treatment of recurrent pterygium. Ann Ophthalmol. 1977; 9(3):352–356

[50] King JH , Jr. The pterygium; brief review and evaluation of certain methods of treatment. AMA Arch Opthalmol. 1950; 44(6):854–869

[51] Hobby CM. An operation for pterygium. Am J Ophthalmol. 1888; 5:94–95

[52] McCoombes JA, Hirst LW, Isbell GP. Sliding conjunctival flap for the treatment of primary pterygium. Ophthalmology. 1994; 101(1):169–173

[53] Hirst LW. The treatment of pterygium. Surv Ophthalmol. 2003; 48(2):145–180

[54] Elschnig HH. Eine neue Rezidivpterygiumoperation. Klin Monatsbl Augenheilkd. 1926; 76:714–716

[55] Sangwan VS, Sharp JAH. Simple limbal epithelial transplantation. Curr Opin Ophthalmol. 2017; 28(4):382–386

[56] Hernández-Bogantes E, Amescua G, Navas A, et al. Minor ipsilateral simple limbal epithelial transplantation (mini-SLET) for pterygium treatment. Br J Ophthalmol. 2015; 99 (12):1598–1600

[57] Stephenson AJ, Griffiths RW, La Hausse-Brown TP. Patterns of contraction in human full thickness skin grafts. Br J Plast Surg. 2000; 53(5):397–402

[58] Gómez-Márquez J.. Un nuevo procedimiento operatorio contra el pterigion. Archivos oftalmologicos Hisp-Amer. 1931; 31:87–95

[59] Duverger C. Extirpation du ptérygion et greffe de muqueuse buccale. Arch Ophthal. 1926; 43:705–708

[60] Wiener M. Treatment of recurrent pterygium. Am J Ophthalmol. 1928; 11(11):876–878

[61] Ip MH, Chui JJ, Tat L, Coroneo MT. Significance of Fuchs flecks in patients with pterygium/pinguecula: earliest indicator of ultraviolet light damage. Cornea. 2015; 34(12): 1560–1563

[62] Dushku N, Reid TW. Immunohistochemical evidence that human pterygia originate from an invasion of vimentin-expressing altered limbal epithelial basal cells. Curr Eye Res. 1994; 13(7):473–481

[63] Dushku N, John MK, Schultz GS, Reid TW. Pterygia pathogenesis: corneal invasion by matrix metalloproteinase expressing altered limbal epithelial basal cells. Arch Ophthalmol. 2001; 119(5):695–706– Erratum in: Arch Ophthalmol. 2002;120:234–7

[64] Jaworski CJ, Aryankalayil-John M, Campos MM, et al. Expression analysis of human pterygium shows a predominance of conjunctival and limbal markers and genes associated with cell migration. Mol Vis. 2009; 15:2421–2434

[65] Coroneo MT. Albedo concentration in the anterior eye: a phenomenon that locates some solar diseases. Ophthalmic Surg. 1990; 21(1):60–66

[66] Coroneo MT. Pterygium as an early indicator of ultraviolet insolation: a hypothesis. Br J Ophthalmol. 1993; 77(11): 734–739

[67] Tagle RB. A new operative technic of conjunctival grafting in the pterygium. Arch Ophthalmol. 1947; 38(3):409

[68] Barraquer JI. Plastias Conjuntivales; Estudios e Informaciones Oftalmológicas. Barcelona, España: Instituto Barraquer; 1948:1(10)

[69] Barraquer JI. Etiology, pathogenesis, and treatment of the pterygium. Symposium on Medical and Surgical Diseases of the Cornea. Transactions of the New Orleans Academy of Ophthalmology. St Louis: CV Mosby; 1980:167–178

[70] Davanger M, Evensen A. Role of the pericorneal papillary structure in renewal of corneal epithelium. Nature. 1971; 229(5286):560–561

[71] Thoft RA, Friend J. The X, Y, Z hypothesis of corneal epithelial maintenance. [letter]. Invest Ophthalmol Vis Sci. 1983; 24(10):1442–1443

[72] Schermer A, Galvin S, Sun TT. Differentiation-related expression of a major 64K corneal keratin in vivo and in culture suggests limbal location of corneal epithelial stem cells. J Cell Biol. 1986; 103(1):49–62

[73] Kenyon KR, Wagoner MD, Hettinger ME. Conjunctival autograft transplantation for advanced and recurrent pterygium. Ophthalmology. 1985; 92(11):1461–1470

[74] Kenyon KR, Tseng SCG. Limbal autograft transplantation for ocular surface disorders. Ophthalmology. 1989; 96(5):709–722, discussion 722–723

[75] Majo F, Rochat A, Nicolas M, Jaoudé GA, Barrandon Y. Oligopotent stem cells are distributed throughout the mammalian ocular surface. Nature. 2008; 456(7219):250–254

[76] Sun TT, Tseng SC, Lavker RM. Location of corneal epithelial stem cells. Nature. 2010; 463(7284):E10–E11, discussion E11

[77] Qi H, Zheng X, Yuan X, Pflugfelder SC, Li DQ. Potential localization of putative stem/progenitor cells in human bulbar conjunctival epithelium. J Cell Physiol. 2010; 225(1):180–185

[78] Güler M, Sobaci G, Ilker S, Oztürk F, Mutlu FM, Yildirim E. Limbal-conjunctival autograft transplantation in cases with recurrent pterygium. Acta Ophthalmol (Copenh). 1994; 72(6):721–726

[79] Gris O, Güell JL, del Campo Z. Limbal-conjunctival autograft transplantation for the treatment of recurrent pterygium. Ophthalmology. 2000; 107(2):270–273

[80] Mejía LF, Sánchez JG, Escobar H. Management of primary pterygia using free conjunctival and limbal-conjunctival autografts without antimetabolites. Cornea. 2005; 24(8):972–975

[81] Han SB, Hyon JY, Hwang JM, Wee WR. Efficacy and safety of limbal-conjunctival autografting with limbal fixation sutures after pterygium excision. Ophthalmologica. 2012; 227(4):210–214

[82] Al Fayez MF. Limbal versus conjunctival autograft transplantation for advanced and recurrent pterygium. Ophthalmology. 2002; 109(9):1752–1755

[83] Al Fayez MF. Limbal-conjunctival vs conjunctival autograft transplant for recurrent pterygia: a prospective randomized controlled trial. JAMA Ophthalmol. 2013; 131(1):11–16

[84] Young AL, Ho M, Jhanji V, Cheng LL. Ten-year results of a randomized controlled trial comparing 0.02% mitomycin C and limbal conjunctival autograft in pterygium surgery. Ophthalmology. 2013; 120(12):2390–2395

[85] Chan TC, Wong RL, Li EY, et al. Twelve-year outcomes of pterygium excision with conjunctival autograft versus intra-operative mitomycin C in double-head pterygium surgery. J Ophthalmol. 2015; 2015:891582

[86] Coroneo MT. Beheading the pterygium. Ophthalmic Surg. 1992; 23(10):691–692

[87] Di Girolamo N, Chui J, Wakefield D, Coroneo MT. Cultured human ocular surface epithelium on therapeutic contact lenses. Br J Ophthalmol. 2007; 91(4):459–464

[88] Goktas S, Sakarya Y, Ozcimen M, et al. Effect of topical cyclopentolate on post-operative pain after pterygium surgery. Clin Exp Optom. 2017; 100(6):595–597

[89] Assaad NN, Chong R, Tat LT, Bennett MH, Coroneo MT. Use of adjuvant hyperbaric oxygen therapy to support limbal conjunctival graft in the management of recurrent pterygium. Cornea. 2011; 30(1):7–10

[90] Sridhar MS, Vemuganti GK, Bansal AK, Rao GN. Impression cytology-proven corneal stem cell deficiency in patients after surgeries involving the limbus. Cornea. 2001; 20(2):145–148

[91] Meallet MA, Espana EM, Grueterich M, Ti SE, Goto E, Tseng SC. Amniotic membrane transplantation with conjunctival limbal autograft for total limbal stem cell deficiency. Ophthalmology. 2003; 110(8):1585–1592

[92] Kim EC, Jun AS, Kim MS, Jee D. Mooren ulcer occurring at donor site after contralateral conjunctivolimbal autograft for recurrent pterygium. Cornea. 2012; 31(11):1357–1358

[93] Tan J, Krilis M Vollmer-Conna U et al. Dry eye disease in recurrent pterygium. Ophthalmic Res 2018 (in press)

[94] Hirst LW. Mitomycin C in the treatment of pterygium. Clin Experiment Ophthalmol. 2006; 34(3):197–198

[95] Hirst LW, Sebban A, Chant D. Pterygium recurrence time. Ophthalmology. 1994; 101(4):755–758

[96] Lin CP, Shih MH, Tsai MC. Clinical experiences of infectious scleral ulceration: a complication of pterygium operation. Br J Ophthalmol. 1997; 81(11):980–983

[97] Doshi RR, Harocopos GJ, Schwab IR, Cunningham ET , Jr. The spectrum of postoperative scleral necrosis. Surv Ophthalmol. 2013; 58(6):620–633

[98] Kim TJ, Choi HJ, Kim MK, Wee WR. Prophylactic removal and microbiological evaluation of calcified plaques after pterygium surgery. Graefes Arch Clin Exp Ophthalmol. 2016; 254(3):553–559

[99] Assaad NN, Coroneo MT. Conjunctival autograft failure in eyes previously exposed to beta-radiation or mitomycin. Arch Ophthalmol. 2008; 126(10):1460–1461

[100] Cameron ME. Pterygium Throughout the World. Springfield, IL: Thomas; 1965

[101] Smith S, D'Amore PA, Dreyer EB. Comparative toxicity of mitomycin C and 5-fluorouracil in vitro. Am J Ophthalmol. 1994; 118(3):332–337

[102] Chan CM, Chew PT, Alsagoff Z, Wong JS, Tan DT. Vascular patterns in pterygium and conjunctival autografting: a pilot study using indocyanine green anterior segment angiography. Br J Ophthalmol. 2001; 85(3):350–353

[103] Perrins DJ. Influence of hyperbaric oxygen on the survival of split skin grafts. Lancet. 1967; 1(7495):868–871

[104] Bowersox JC, Strauss MB, Hart GB. Clinical experience with hyperbaric oxygen therapy in the salvage of ischemic skin flaps and grafts. J Hyperbaric Med.. 1986; 1:141–149

[105] Tan JCK, Kuo MX, Coroneo MT. Autoconjunctival graft compromise after pterygium surgery in a patient receiving intravitreal anti-vascular endothelial growth factor injections. Cornea. 2016; 35(12):1653–1655

[106] Van Geest RJ, Lesnik-Oberstein SY, Tan HS, et al. A shift in the balance of vascular endothelial growth factor and connective tissue growth factor by bevacizumab causes the

angiofibrotic switch in proliferative diabetic retinopathy. Br J Ophthalmol. 2012; 96(4):587–590

[107] Zhang F, Lineaweaver W. Acute and sustained effects of vascular endothelial growth factor on survival of flaps and skin grafts. Ann Plast Surg. 2011; 66(5):581–582

[108] Vrabec MP, Weisenthal RW, Elsing SH. Subconjunctival fibrosis after conjunctival autograft. Cornea. 1993; 12(2):181–183

[109] Shimazaki J, Shinozaki N, Tsubota K. Transplantation of amniotic membrane and limbal autograft for patients with recurrent pterygium associated with symblepharon. Br J Ophthalmol. 1998; 82(3):235–240

[110] Hirst LW. Pterygium removal using a polyethylene glycol hydrogel adherent ocular bandage. Cornea. 2013; 32(6):803–805

[111] Suprachoroidal Drainage – Centenarian Progress: An Inventor's Perspective. In: Francis BA, Sarkisian S Tan J, eds. Minimally Invasive Glaucoma Surgery: the Science and the Practice. New York: Thieme; 2016

[112] Lu L, Xu S, Ge S, et al. Tailored treatment for the management of scleral necrosis following pterygium excision. Exp Ther Med. 2017; 13(3):845–850

[113] Yoshida M, Yokokura S, Kunikata H, et al. Endophthalmitis associated with Purpureocillium lilacinum during infliximab treatment for surgically induced necrotizing scleritis, successfully treated with 27-gauge vitrectomy. Int Ophthalmol. 2018; 38(2):841–847

[114] Krilis M, Tsang H, Coroneo M. Treatment of conjunctival and corneal epithelial neoplasia with retinoic acid and topical interferon alfa-2b: long-term follow-up. Ophthalmology. 2012; 119(10):1969–1973

[115] Oke I, Alkharashi M, Petersen RA, Ashenberg A, Shah AS. Treatment of Ocular Pyogenic Granuloma With Topical Timolol. JAMA Ophthalmol. 2017; 135(4):383–385

[116] Kuo MX, Sarris M, Coroneo MT. Cadaveric porcine model for teaching and practicing conjunctival autograft creation. Cornea. 2015; 34(7):824–828

[117] Zhang X, Li Q, Liu B, et al. In vivo cross-sectional observation and thickness measurement of bulbar conjunctiva using optical coherence tomography. Invest Ophthalmol Vis Sci. 2011; 52(10):7787–7791

[118] Trikha S, Turnbull AM, Morris RJ, Anderson DF, Hossain P. The journey to femtosecond laser-assisted cataract surgery: new beginnings or a false dawn? Eye (Lond). 2013; 27(4):461–473

[119] Pahlitzsch M, Torun N, Pahlitzsch ML, et al. Impact of the femtosecond laser in line with the femtosecond laser-assisted cataract surgery (FLACS) on the anterior chamber characteristics in comparison to the manual phacoemulsification. Semin Ophthalmol. 2017; 32(4):456–461

[120] Soong HK, Malta JB. Femtosecond lasers in ophthalmology. Am J Ophthalmol. 2009; 147(2):189–197.e2

[121] Zhou Y, Zhang J, Tian L, Zhai C. Comparison of the Ziemer FEMTO LDV femtosecond laser and Moria M2 mechanical microkeratome. J Refract Surg. 2012; 28(3):189–194

[122] Santhiago MR, Kara-Junior N, Waring GO , IV. Microkeratome versus femtosecond flaps: accuracy and complications. Curr Opin Ophthalmol. 2014; 25(4):270–274

[123] Fuest M, Liu YC, Yam GH, et al. Femtosecond laser-assisted conjunctival autograft preparation for pterygium surgery. Ocul Surf. 2017; 15(2):211–217

[124] Fuest M, Liu YC, Coroneo MT, Mehta JS. Femtosecond Laser Assisted Pterygium Surgery. Cornea. 2017; 36(7):889–892

[125] Fuest M, Mehta JS, Coroneo MT. New treatment options for pterygium. Editorial. Expert Rev Ophthalmol. 2017; 12(3):193–196

[126] de Medeiros FW, Kaur H, Agrawal V, et al. Effect of femtosecond laser energy level on corneal stromal cell death and inflammation. J Refract Surg. 2009; 25(10):869–874

[127] Calcagni M, Althaus MK, Knapik AD, et al. In vivo visualization of the origination of skin graft vasculature in a wild-type/GFP crossover model. Microvasc Res. 2011; 82(3):237–245

8 Amniotic Graft Surgery in Ocular Surface Pathologies besides Pterygium

Arun C. Gulani

Abstract

Amniotic grafts can be used in a full-spectrum ocular surface and corneal disorders for aesthetically and visually excellent outcomes. Such disorders include corneal surface instability, recurrent corneal erosions, Lasik complications, Salzmann's nodules, and anterior corneal dystrophies.

Keywords: pterygium surgery, ProKera, corneal scars, Lasik complications, Intacs, Keratoconus, corneal dystrophy

8.1 Introduction

Having always approached pterygium surgery as a corneal and ocular surface pathology allowed me to extend this surgical technique to various other associated and nonassociated corneal and ocular surface pathologies successfully, and in many cases, result in more than cosmetic outcomes to even enhancing function as a vision endpoint.[1]

I shall share my experience in this category with various such pathologies, especially presenting this surgical concept as a least invasive and easily adaptable surgery with corneal transplant and other relatively more invasive surgeries as backup.[2,3]

8.2 Band-Shaped Keratopathy

In cases with band-shaped keratopathy (BSK), many patients had come to terms with their irreversibly blind eyes, but suffered from poor cosmetic appearances and hence low self-esteem. Still, they did not want an invasive cosmetic corneal transplant.

I approached these cases like a corneal pathology, and on lifting the BSK calcific plaques, I was surprised to see in majority of cases a smooth stromal base that could be draped with the amniotic graft centrally and be secured with glue in addition to a single perilimbal suture for a long-term application on these uneven corneal shapes to excellent cosmetic outcomes.

In all cases, I used mitomycin C 0.04% for 30 seconds prior to application of amniotic graft. Three cases had a recurrence of their BSK, but much less than that at preoperative levels, and patients appreciated the near-normal cosmetic appearance of their operated eyes.

Prototype of BSK cases are explained in ▶ Fig. 8.1, ▶ Fig. 8.2, ▶ Fig. 8.3.

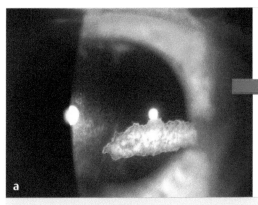
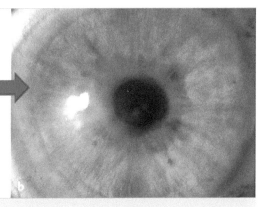

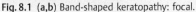
Fig. 8.1 (a,b) Band-shaped keratopathy: focal.

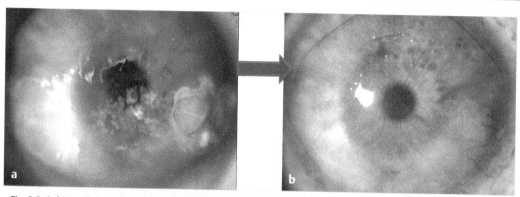

Fig. 8.2 (a,b) Band-shaped keratopathy: diffuse.

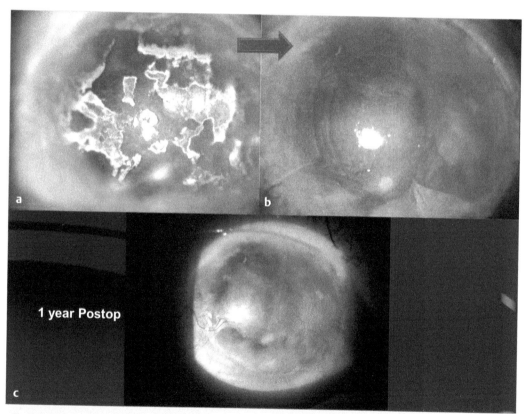

Fig. 8.3 (a-c) Focal band-shaped keratopathy.

8.3 Restoring and Rejuvenating Non-Healing Corneal Surface

In cases with delayed epithelial healing, especially from neuropathy and ocular surface instability (▶ Fig. 8.4 and ▶ Fig. 8.5), I have found amniotic graft application to be especially useful not only as a less invasive surgical approach but also as a cosmetically oriented endeavor.

In some cases, adherence of graft was achieved with Tisseel glue (most of these had normal corneal contour), while in some (with irregular corneal shapes), I always applied a single, perilimbal 10–0 nylon suture.

I have used it for cases of anterior and posterior corneal surgery stabilization including in cases such as shown in ▶ Fig. 8.6 where poor anterior corneal healing led to a patient being dissatisfied with his surgeon despite a well-done Descemet stripping automated endothelial keratoplasty (DSAEK) surgery and on anterior clearance with amniotic membrane transplantation (AMT) recovered vision and optical clarity.

8.4 ProKera

Amniotic membrane in a bandage contact lens is a modality that can help heal the ocular surface as

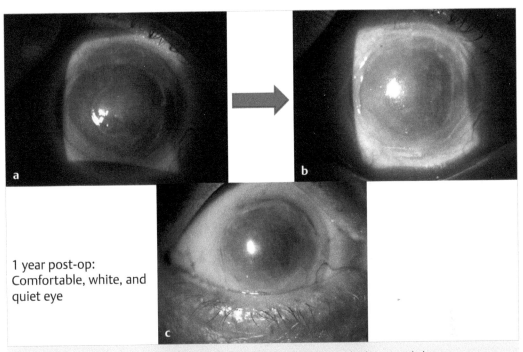

1 year post-op: Comfortable, white, and quiet eye

Fig. 8.4 (a-c) Amniotic membrane transplantation (AMT) for neurotrophic non-healing corneal ulcer.

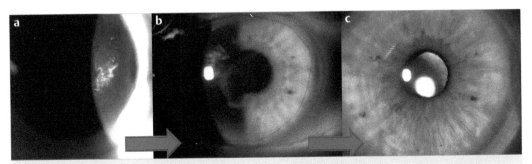

Fig. 8.5 (a-c) Amniotic membrane transplantation (AMT) for corneal scar with recurrent corneal erosion (RCE).

well as decrease associated inflammation and restore surface stability in numerous cases, where I have used it for refractive complications, that were referred to me for reasons of poor healing or complications limited to surface corneal issues.

In associated images, you can see applications in Lasik epithelial ingrowth, Intacs wound healing, corneal dystrophy, corneal scars and irregularities, non-healing corneal surface post laser Corneoplastique for corneal scars, preoperatively to prepare

ocular surface for laser correction of corneal irregularities, etc. (▶ Fig. 8.7, ▶ Fig. 8.8, ▶ Fig. 8.9, ▶ Fig. 8.10, ▶ Fig. 8.11, ▶ Fig. 8.12, ▶ Fig. 8.13, ▶ Fig. 8.14, ▶ Fig. 8.15, ▶ Fig. 8.16).

I have also used this modality in very irregular and flat corneas (such as some with extremely low keratometry and dense corneal scar removals) immediately post laser treatments since normal bandage contact lenses (BLC) would not stay on such corneas.

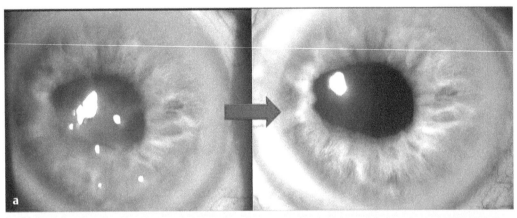

Fig. 8.6 (a,b) Amniotic membrane transplantation (AMT) for Descemet stripping automated endothelial keratoplasty (DSAEK) with corneal scar.

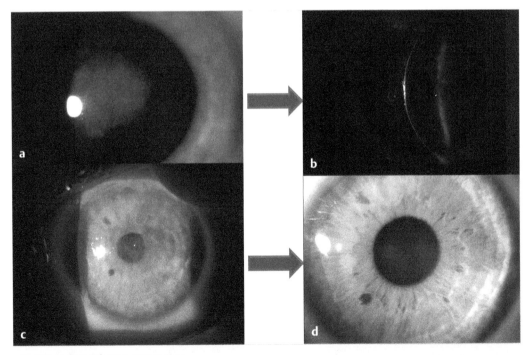

Fig. 8.7 (a-d) CL infection scar: ProKera.

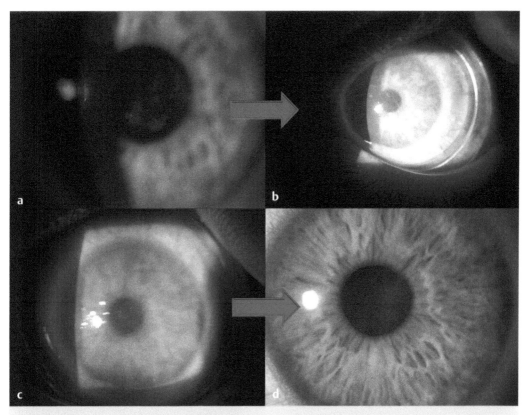

Fig. 8.8 (a-d) Photorefractive keratectomy (PRK) scar: ProKera.

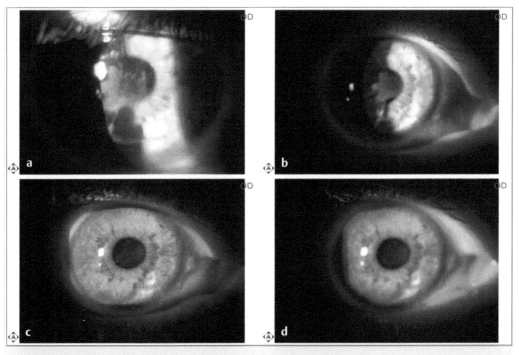

Fig. 8.9 (a-d) Radial keratotomy (RK) scar: Lamellar keratectomy (LK) + ProKera.

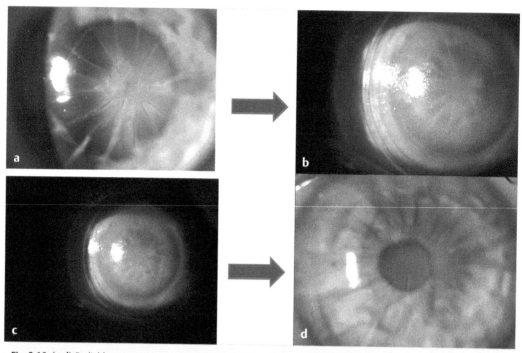

Fig. 8.10 (a-d) Radial keratotomy scars: laser Corneoplastique + ProKera.

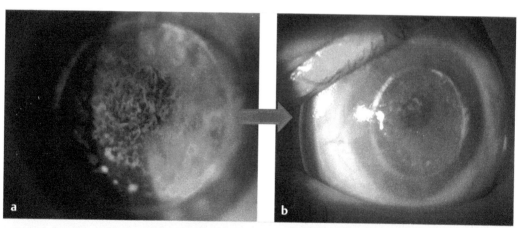

Fig. 8.11 (a,b) Corneal dystrophy: Lamellar keratectomy (LK) + Prokera.

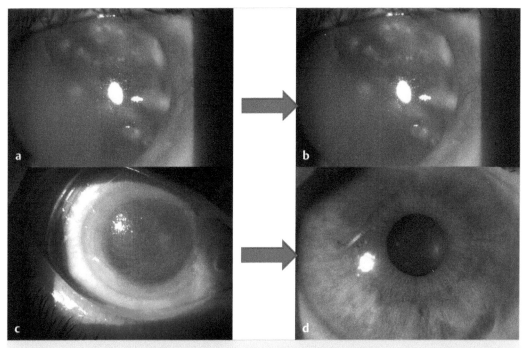

Fig. 8.12 (a-d) Salzmann's nodules: Lamellar keratectomy (LK) + Prokera.

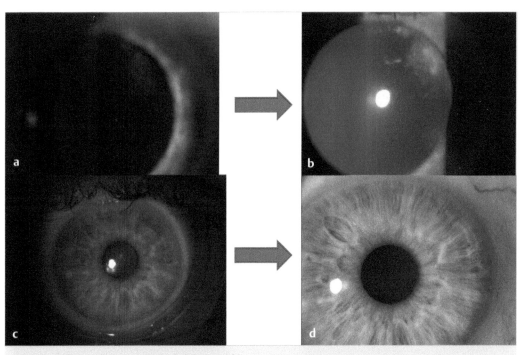

Fig. 8.13 (a-d) Lasik flap scar (s/p epithelial ingrowth).

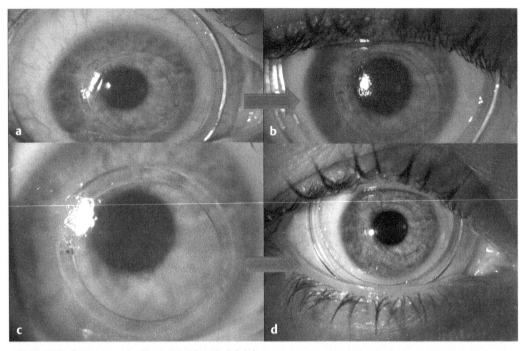

Fig. 8.14 (a-d) Intacs non-healing incisional epithelial defect.

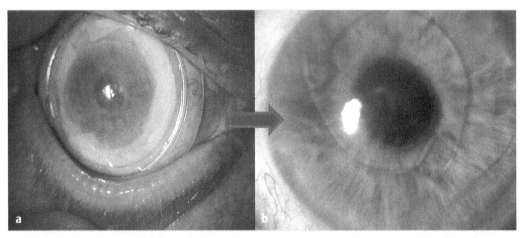

Fig. 8.15 (a,b) Pseudophakic bullous keratopathy: ProKera post Descemet stripping automated endothelial keratoplasty (DSAEK).

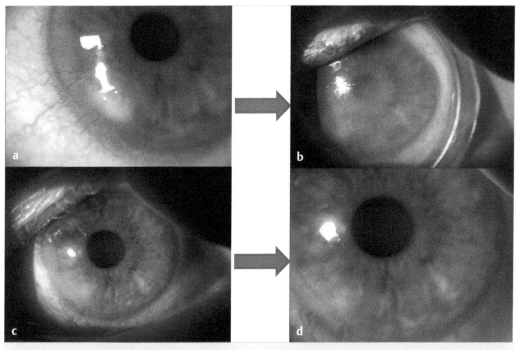

Fig. 8.16 (a-d) Lasik flap edge melt.

8.4.1 Kerato-amnioplasty

In certain cases of corneal non-healing associated with thin and unstable cornea, I have combined amniotic graft application with lamellar keratoplasty.

I have called it kerato-amnioplasty, when done simultaneously where I sutured the amniotic graft while suturing the lamellar cornea graft. (▶ Fig. 8.17).

In some cases, I first performed lamellar keratoplasty and on securing more regular surface, applied the amniotic graft on the top with Tisseel glue at the same surgical sitting, as in ▶ Fig. 8.18 where this patient who was referred with neurotrophic, non-healing corneal ulcer with scar despite a lateral tarsorrhaphy did very well for 7 years with her lamellar keratectomy and sutured AMT at which point her scar returned. You can still see the perilimbal suture from 7 years ago. This patient now underwent a lamellar keratoplasty with glued AMT (▶ Fig. 8.18).

8.5 Amniotic Graft as a Substrate for Stem Cells

Simple limbal stem cell transplant (SLET) involves application of an amniotic graft to the poor corneal surface and using that as a base to then place limbal stem cell transplant pieces on it and secure them with Tisseel glue followed by bandage contact lenses (BCL) placement (▶ Fig. 8.19). ProKera can also be used in such cases.

Thus, amniotic graft—with its transparent properties that are aesthetically appealing, healing properties that are medically appealing, and with its ease of surgical application, including least interventional—is a versatile surgical tool to take care of the entire spectrum of ocular surface and

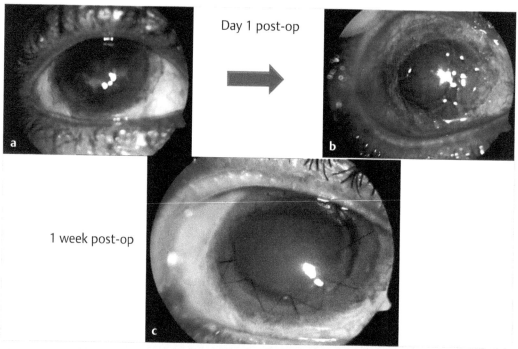

Fig. 8.17 (a-c) Kerato-amnioplasty.

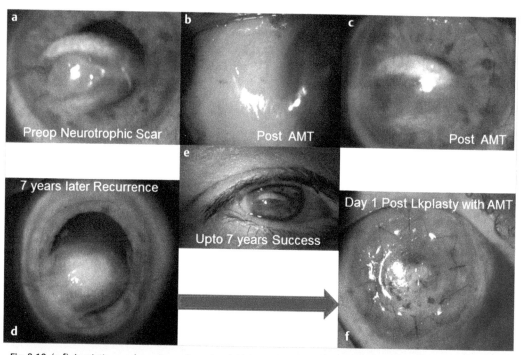

Fig. 8.18 (a-f) Amniotic membrane transplantation (AMT): 7 years later; LKplasty + glued AMT.

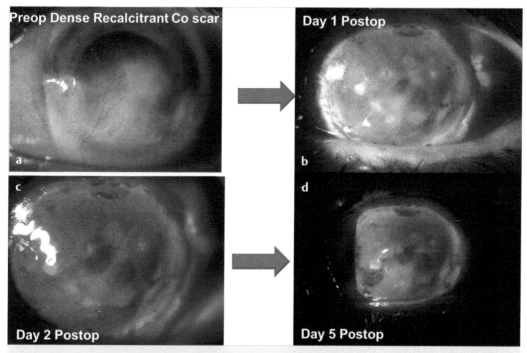

Fig. 8.19 (a-d) Simple limbal stem cell transplant (SLET): amniotic membrane transplantation (AMT) with glued limbal grafts.

corneal pathologies,[4] including various refractive, non-refractive, and surgical conundrums.

References

[1] Gulani AC. Surgical method sets higher standard for managing pterygium. Ocular Surgery News. Consultation Section, Aug 2008

[2] Gulani AC. Pterygium and pinguecula surgery: cosmetic desires for future of ocular surface surgery. Video Journal of Ophthalmology. 2009

[3] Gulani AC. Sutureless amniotic surgery for pterygium: cosmetic outcomes for ocular surface surgery. Tech Ophthalmol. 2008; 6(2):41–44

[4] Gulani AC. A Cornea-friendly pterygium procedure. Rev Ophthalmol. 2012; 18(6):52–56

9 Mitomycin C, Glues, Sealants, and Ancillaries in Pterygium Surgery

Arun C. Gulani and Sonal Tuli

Abstract

Adjunct therapies are frequently used in pterygium surgery to improve outcomes and to prevent recurrences. Sealants and cautery fixation have considerably shortened the time taken to perform the surgery compared to suturing. The various therapies used to decrease the recurrence rate include anti-vascular endothelial growth factor (anti-VEGF) agents, immunomodulatory therapies, and radiation.

Keywords: pterygium surgery, cytostatics, mitomycin, 5-FU, anti-VEGF, cyclosporine, fibrin glue, autologous blood, beta radiation

9.1 Introduction

Over nearly three decades of performing pterygium surgery and constantly honing the technique to cosmetic and yet visually accountable outcomes, I came to realize that many ancillary developments in technology and material were nearly essential to such high expectations in outcomes and safety.

Having observed surgeons and worked with patients from all over the world, it has become clear to me that no two surgeons have an identical surgical approach or philosophy to pterygium, and that no two patients have ever presented with an exactly similar pathology.

The acceptance of this reality in itself leads to this chapter where my coauthor reviews ancillary adjuncts to pterygium surgery and their impact, both negative and positive leaving open a platform for each surgeon to still not change their own time-trusted techniques drastically but maybe encourage a small change along the way.

Pterygium surgery, like cataract surgery, was first described thousands of years ago by Sushruta in India.[1] He described a bare sclera technique of pterygium removal and discussed the fact that improper removal would result in recurrence. However, unlike the spectacular success rate of modern-day cataract surgery compared to his description of couching cataracts, the improvements made in pterygium surgery are relatively modest without exciting breakthroughs. Even in the modern times, it continues to be plagued by high recurrence rates and extended surgical times.

Recurrences after pterygium surgery occur due to regrowth of fibrovascular tissue from the conjunctiva and episclera over the limbus and onto the cornea due to lack of the barrier of the normal limbal stem cells. In the bare sclera method of pterygium surgery, the pterygium is excised, and no further procedures are performed. The fibrovascular tissue peripheral to the pterygium rapidly replicates and grows back over the existing defect, resulting in a recurrent pterygium. However, if the barrier is recreated either by transplanting limbal cells from another area as in a conjunctival limbal autograft (CLAU), or by delaying the growth of the fibrovascular tissue until existing stem cells peripheral to the area of the pterygium expand and cover the defect, the risk of recurrence can be theoretically reduced.

It is well established that CLAU significantly decreases recurrences compared to other methods of pterygium surgery.[2,3] However, harvesting CLAU takes a considerable investment in surgical time, and CLAU is not always possible in cases with extensive scarring, double header, or recurrent pterygia. In these cases, the alternatives include amniotic membrane or buccal mucus membrane transplantation, which have lower recurrence rates than bare sclera has, but still have a much higher recurrence rate than CLAU. Therefore, a large variety of ancillary therapies have been investigated to reduce recurrence rates and to improve surgical times.

9.2 Ancillaries

9.2.1 Cytostatics

Cytostatic medications are used in chemotherapy of cancers to inhibit cell growth. Unlike typical cytotoxic chemotherapeutic agents, such as cyclophosphamide, that kill the tumor cells, these medications work by inhibiting cellular replication. These drugs most commonly used for pterygium surgery are mitomycin C (MMC) and 5-fluorouracil (5-FU). They inhibit cellular replication by inhibiting deoxyribonucleic acid (DNA) synthesis; cells

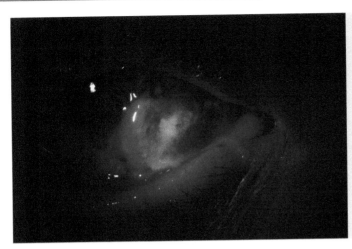

Fig. 9.1 Scleral necrosis following pterygium excision with mitomycin C (MMC) and amniotic membrane transplantation (AMT).

then undergo apoptosis and fibrotic activity is reduced.

9.2.2 Mitomycin C

Mitomycin C (MMC) is an alkylating agent that is derived from *Streptomyces caespitosus*. It has been used in pterygium surgery since the 1960s in Asia, but became popular in the western world since the late 1980s. It inhibits the synthesis of DNA in all cells at all stages of the cell cycle. Cell death from apoptosis occurs, as cells are unable to repair the injury caused by alkylation. In addition, it inhibits messenger ribonucleic acid (mRNA) and has antiangiogenic properties. As it works on all stages of the cell cycle, it is a very potent inhibitor of fibroblast proliferation, collagen deposition, and vasculogenesis. As anticipated, these effects decrease inflammation and fibrovascular proliferation, thus reducing the risk of recurrences after pterygium surgery.[4] In addition, the inhibitive effect of MMC on fibroblast proliferation may also decrease the density of scarring under the head of the pterygium after removal.[5] MMC has been used with the bare sclera technique as well as with autografts and amniotic membrane transplantation (AMT).[6] All the studies attest to its efficacy in reducing recurrences with the possible exception of CLAU surgery in primary pterygia where studies indicate that there may not be any additional benefit to adding MMC, but the adverse events may increase compared to those with CLAU alone.[7]

However, these very same antimitogenic effects also contribute to the risks associated with MMC use. Irritation of the ocular surface and photophobia are common symptoms associated with ptery-gium excision but are exaggerated with the use of MMC. However, MMC use has also been associated with various vision-threatening complications, such as necrotizing scleritis, sterile melts and calcification, corneal ulceration and edema, delayed epithelial healing, and iritis (▶ Fig. 9.1).[8,9,10] The risk of these complications ranges widely and may be related to the concentration of MMC, the duration of its contact with the ocular surface, and the surgery performed (whether bare sclera or grafted). Increasing the dose and duration of MMC, while decreasing the risk of recurrence, increases the risk of complications. Therefore, it would be prudent to use MMC only in high-risk or recurrent cases of pterygium and at the lowest doses possible.

9.2.3 Intraoperative

Using MMC intraoperatively is the most common technique used in literature. MMC is usually applied in concentrations between 0.02 and 0.05% after the pterygium is excised.[3,6] It is usually applied using a soaked sponge either to the bare sclera or to the Tenon's capsule surrounding the excised area. It is kept in situ for 3 to 5 minutes and is thoroughly washed out with balanced salt solution. The advantage of this method is that it is easy to use and is able to be titrated to some extent by modifying the concentration and duration. There is a plethora of articles in literature attesting to the efficacy of MMC in preventing recurrences in primary as well as recurrent pterygia, and it is a well-established adjunct to pterygium surgery. However, it is associated with all the complications of MMC, including scleral melts and ocular surface toxicity.[11]

9.2.4 Preoperative MMC

The disadvantage of intraoperative MMC is that the actual dose of MMC that the eye is exposed to is unpredictable. Preoperative MMC has the advantage that the exact total dose of MMC can be precisely titrated. In this method, MMC is injected under the head of the pterygium, at various times ranging from a month prior to the day before surgery.[12,13] However, studies have not found a significant difference in either the efficacy or the adverse events with this modality as compared to intraoperative application and is not used widely.[14]

9.2.5 Postoperative MMC

The first reports of using MMC for pterygium surgery used the postoperative, topical approach.[15] The drops were started either immediately or approximately a month following surgery. Although the recurrence rates of topical MMC are similar to intraoperative MMC, the complications are significantly higher, and this method is not recommended currently. There is a single report of using a single-drop topical MMC immediately post surgery with similar reduction in recurrence as intraoperative, but lower risk of complications such as scleral necrosis and epithelial toxicity.[16]

9.2.6 5-Fluorouracil

5-FU is a pyrimidine analog that inhibits DNA synthesis in the S phase of the mitotic cycle and, therefore, primarily prevents replication of rapidly proliferating cells only. It is thus a much weaker inhibitor of pterygium recurrence.[17] It has similar side effects as MMC and is, therefore, used much less commonly with pterygium surgery.[17]

9.2.7 Anti-vascular Endothelial Growth Factor Agents

Vascular endothelial growth factor (VEGF) has been found in abundance in pterygium tissue leading to the speculation that it has an etiological role in the development of pterygia.[18] In addition, higher levels of VEGF in pterygium excision specimens have been found to correlate to more significant recurrences.[18] Therefore, logic suggests that the use of anti-VEGF drugs may be beneficial in reducing recurrences after pterygium surgery. Bevacizumab is the most commonly studied anti-VEGF agent used in pterygium surgery. It is typically injected into the pterygium prior to surgery or used postoperatively either as an injection or topical drops.[19,20] Unfortunately, the results have been mixed with some studies indicating a significant reduction in recurrences with a much better safety profile than MMC, while others have found no significant effect.[21,22] Subconjunctival injections of anti-VEGF agents for recurrent pterygia also had similar mixed results. While some studies showed that there was a reduction in the vascularity and size of recurrent pterygia, others showed that the effect was only temporary and increased back to baseline a few weeks later.[23,24]

9.2.8 Cyclosporine

Cyclosporine A (CsA) was initially isolated from the filamentous fungus *Tolypocladium inflatum* as an antifungal agent by Sandoz. However, it was soon found to be a potent anti-inflammatory and immunosuppressant agent and is used widely to prevent transplant rejection. These immunomodulatory effects have led to its widespread use in ophthalmology and ocular surface disorders, such as dry eye and vernal keratoconjunctivitis. Recently, there have been several reports of its use in preventing pterygium recurrence. Its mechanism of action is thought to be its binding to T-lymphocytes and inhibiting calcineurin. This, in turn, inhibits the inflammatory cascade mediated by matrix metalloproteinases that breaks down the collagen and stimulates the production of fibroblasts and vasculature.

Unfortunately, CsA is a large molecular weight hydrophobic molecule that does not dissolve in aqueous solutions. Therefore, commonly available commercial CsA formulations are nanoemulsions (Restasis in the United States and Ikervis in the European Union). They are both approved for the treatment of dry eye, and their use in pterygia is off-label. CsA is useful in pterygia as it is an effective inhibitor of pterygium fibroblasts and, additionally, endothelial cell proliferation and angiogenesis.

A prospective study of 31 patients with bilateral pterygia was conducted by Yalcin Tok et al.[25] All pterygia were removed using the bare sclera technique. Subsequently, one eye of each patient had been assigned to postoperative topical CsA (Restasis) for 6 months, while the fellow eyes served as controls. They found that the pterygium recurred in 13% of the CsA eyes, while 45% of the control eyes had recurrence of pterygia. Other randomized controlled studies have shown similar improve-

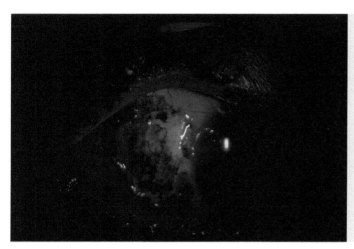

Fig. 9.2 Glued autograft with mild retraction of nasal margin.

ments in the recurrence rates with the bare sclera as well as conjunctival flap techniques.[26,27]

9.2.9 Sealants

Fibrin Glue

The use of fibrin to close ocular wounds is not new. In 1950, Tassman[28] and Town and Naidoff[29] simultaneously published reports describing the use of fibrin glue to close conjunctival wounds as well as cataract surgery wounds. They used either autologous plasma or commercially available plasma and reconstituted, commercially available thrombin. They found that the wound closure was immediate and stable. It was used in pterygium surgery in the 1990s along with sutures, but it was only when fibrin glue became commercially available that it was used widely for fixation of grafts in pterygium surgery. Tisseel and Evicel are two of the commercially available fibrin-based sealants used routinely in surgery.[30] They are both made from pooled plasma and consist of two components, fibrinogen and thrombin, which are mixed together to make a fibrin clot.

Fibrin sealants are now a well-established method for fixing both CLAU as well as AMT during pterygium surgery. Randomized controlled studies have shown that fibrin sealants significantly decrease the surgical time, and the risk of recurrence is as low as, or lower than in suture fixation.[31,32] The rationale behind this is that the immediate adherence of the graft results in lower fibroblast activity and less inflammation. However, the complication rate is higher too, with the major complication being graft dehiscence and graft loss

(▶ Fig. 9.2). Additionally, there is a theoretical risk of transmission of blood-borne diseases.

To minimize the risk of disease transmission, autologous fibrin glue can be made by centrifuging and cryoprecipitating the patient's own blood.[33] However, since this is time consuming, it has to be made in advance of the surgery and requires the surgeon to have the necessary equipment for manufacturing it in a sterile environment. It has similar efficacy and complications as commercial fibrin glue has.[34]

9.2.10 Autologous Blood

Although fibrin glue has many advantages, it has significant disadvantages too. Since it is made from pooled plasma, there is a theoretical risk of transmitting infectious diseases. Patients may get sensitized to the foreign proteins in the glue and get an allergic response. There have been reports of anaphylactic reactions to the glue. In addition, fibrin glue is very expensive, storage can be challenging, and the process for mixing and applying can be time consuming and messy. Generating autologous fibrin is time consuming and not practical for eye surgery.

A cheap and quick alternative to fibrin sealants is autologous blood. Using the patient's own blood eliminates the risk of transmitting disease via blood products. Typically, the procedure is performed by placing the graft over a scleral bed that has been either minimally cauterized or not cauterized at all to allow blood to pool under the graft. The graft is then held in position until the blood coagulates, and pressure is applied to tamponade the bleeding vessels so that excessive blood does not collect under the graft.

Multiple prospective and retrospective studies have compared autologous blood and fibrin glue. A prospective randomized study comparing sutures, fibrin glue, and autologous blood coagulum (ABC) found that the time taken to perform the surgery was statistically shorter with ABC compared to the other two techniques.[35] Unfortunately, nearly every study has shown that the risk of graft dehiscence and graft loss is very high with ABC compared to all other techniques of graft adhesion.[32,36] The majority of the studies on ABC have been conducted in developing nations, such as India; it is rare to see ABC used in developed nations.

ReSure

I have also used ReSure sealant in some pterygium cases that needed extensive surgery and additionally in some cases that were traveling back to their out of state and country destinations after surgery for additional protection.

ReSure sealant (Ocular Therapeutix) is a synthetic sealant composed of a polyethylene glycol hydrogel. It comes as two separate materials, a polyethylene glycol solution and a trilysine amine solution, that form a sealant when mixed together. It is Food and Drug Administration (FDA) approved for sealing cataract wounds, but has been used off-label for pterygium surgery.

A retrospective study of nine eyes of seven patients who underwent pterygium excision with AMT and ReSure showed that it was safe and effective with no dislocations or recurrences.

Fixation by Cautery

Another technique that has been described to fix pterygia is using the electrocautery pen (ECP).[37,38]

In this technique, the graft is "welded" to the conjunctival edges at regular intervals using ECP. Studies showed that this technique was superior to sutures and fibrin glue in terms of discomfort for the patient. However, recurrence rate and dislocation are issues with this technique too, and it has not found much favor.

9.2.11 Steroids

Inflammation after pterygium surgery is a known, potent trigger of recurrences. Therefore, steroids are routinely used topically after pterygium excision. Studies have evaluated the role of injecting a long-acting steroid in addition immediately following pterygium excision on recurrences, but the results have been underwhelming with minimal efficacy.[39,40] Studies have also evaluated injecting long-acting steroids, such as triamcinolone, in impending recurrences and have found that it does decrease the risk of recurrences more than topical steroids alone.[41] However, the risks of steroid induced glaucoma must be considered as the sub-Tenon steroids cannot be easily removed in case increased intraocular pressure develops.

9.2.12 Radiation

Beta irradiation has been used as a method to prevent pterygium recurrence since the 1950s. Strontium 90 (Sr90) is the most commonly used source of radiation and is applied to the bed of the pterygium following surgery, although external beam radiation and other modalities have also been used. While studies have universally found that this therapy is effective in reducing recurrences with low immediate adverse effects, long-term studies have shown that late complications of this modality can be very significant (▶ Fig. 9.3).[42,43,44]

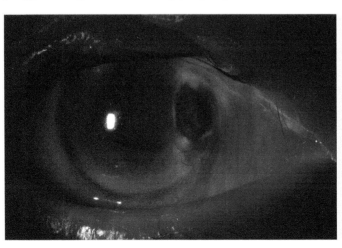

Fig. 9.3 Corneal melt 20 years following pterygium removal with radiation.

Scleromalacia, eyelid adhesion, and scleral ulceration can be seen decades after the procedure and lead to loss of vision in the eye from endophthalmitis.[42,45] This modality is rarely used currently.

Our quest for pterygium surgery to reach heights of safety, zero recurrence, and result in sparkling eyes with emmetropic vision outcomes underscores the need to keep discovering ancillaries that make it more reproducible in all surgical hands and patients alike.

References

[1] Raju VK. Susruta of ancient India. Indian J Ophthalmol. 2003; 51(2):119–122

[2] Chan TC, Wong RL, Li EY, et al. Twelve-year outcomes of pterygium excision with conjunctival autograft versus intraoperative mitomycin C in double-head pterygium surgery. J Ophthalmol. 2015; 2015:891582

[3] Kaufman SC, Jacobs DS, Lee WB, Deng SX, Rosenblatt MI, Shtein RM. Options and adjuvants in surgery for pterygium: a report by the American Academy of Ophthalmology. Ophthalmology. 2013; 120(1):201–208

[4] da Costa Paula C, Julio G, Campos P, Pujol P, Asaad M. Effects of mitomycin c in early conjunctival inflammation after pterygium surgery. Curr Eye Res. 2017; 42(5):696–700

[5] Kam KW, Kwok RP, Belin MW, Young AL. Long-Term density changes in corneal layers after primary pterygium excision with topical mitomycin-C. Cornea. 2016; 35(8):1093–1096

[6] Martins TG, Costa AL, Alves MR, Chammas R, Schor P. Mitomycin C in pterygium treatment. Int J Ophthalmol. 2016; 9 (3):465–468

[7] Long T, Li Z. Bare sclera resection followed by mitomycin C and/or autograft limbus conjunctiva in the surgery for pterygium: a meta-analysis. Int J Ophthalmol. 2015; 8(5):1067–1073

[8] Lindquist TP, Lee WB. Mitomycin C-associated scleral stromalysis after pterygium surgery. Cornea. 2015; 34(4):398–401

[9] Zhivov A, Beck R, Guthoff RF. Corneal and conjunctival findings after mitomycin C application in pterygium surgery: an in-vivo confocal microscopy study. Acta Ophthalmol. 2009; 87(2):166–172

[10] Garcia-Medina JJ, Del-Rio-Vellosillo M, Zanon-Moreno V, Ortiz-Gomariz A, Morcillo-Guardiola M, Pinazo-Duran MD. Severe scleral dellen as an early complication of pterygium excision with simple conjunctival closure and review of the literature. Arq Bras Oftalmol. 2014; 77(3):182–184

[11] Tsai YY, Lin JM, Shy JD. Acute scleral thinning after pterygium excision with intraoperative mitomycin C: a case report of scleral dellen after bare sclera technique and review of the literature. Cornea. 2002; 21(2):227–229

[12] Donnenfeld ED, Perry HD, Fromer S, Doshi S, Solomon R, Biser S. Subconjunctival mitomycin C as adjunctive therapy before pterygium excision. Ophthalmology. 2003; 110(5):1012–1016

[13] Lee DH, Cho HJ, Kim JT, Choi JS, Joo CK. Expression of vascular endothelial growth factor and inducible nitric oxide synthase in pterygia. Cornea. 2001; 20(7):738–742

[14] Zaky KS, Khalifa YM. Efficacy of preoperative injection versus intraoperative application of mitomycin in recurrent pterygium surgery. Indian J Ophthalmol. 2012; 60(4):273–276

[15] Singh G, Wilson MR, Foster CS. Mitomycin eye drops as treatment for pterygium. Ophthalmology. 1988; 95(6):813–821

[16] Gupta VP, Saxena T. Comparison of single-drop mitomycin C regime with other mitomycin C regimes in pterygium surgery. Indian J Ophthalmol. 2003; 51(1):59–65

[17] Kareem AA, Farhood QK, Alhammami HA. The use of antimetabolites as adjunctive therapy in the surgical treatment of pterygium. Clin Ophthalmol. 2012; 6:1849–1854

[18] Gumus K, Karakucuk S, Mirza GE, Akgun H, Arda H, Oner AO. Overexpression of vascular endothelial growth factor receptor 2 in pterygia may have a predictive value for a higher postoperative recurrence rate. Br J Ophthalmol. 2014; 98(6):796–800

[19] Nuzzi R, Tridico F. Efficacy of subconjunctival bevacizumab injections before and after surgical excision in preventing pterygium recurrence. J Ophthalmol. 2017; 2017:6824670

[20] Kasetsuwan N, Reinprayoon U, Satitpitakul V. Prevention of recurrent pterygium with topical bevacizumab 0.05% eye drops: a randomized controlled trial. Clin Ther. 2015; 37(10):2347–2351

[21] Liu J, Xu JH, Xu W, et al. Bevacizumab as adjuvant therapy in the management of pterygium: a systematic review and Meta-analysis. Int J Ophthalmol. 2017; 10(7):1126–1133

[22] Singh P, Sarkar L, Sethi HS, Gupta VS. A randomized controlled prospective study to assess the role of subconjunctival bevacizumab in primary pterygium surgery in Indian patients. Indian J Ophthalmol. 2015; 63(10):779–784

[23] Stival LR, Lago AM, Figueiredo MN, Bittar RH, Machado ML, Nassaralla Junior JJ. Efficacy and safety of subconjunctival bevacizumab for recurrent pterygium. Arq Bras Oftalmol. 2014; 77(1):4–7

[24] Lekhanont K, Patarakittam T, Thongphiew P, Suwan-apichon O, Hanutsaha P. Randomized controlled trial of subconjunctival bevacizumab injection in impending recurrent pterygium: a pilot study. Cornea. 2012; 31(2):155–161

[25] Yalcin Tok O, Burcu Nurozler A, Ergun G, Akbas Kocaoglu F, Duman S. Topical cyclosporine A in the prevention of pterygium recurrence. Ophthalmologica. 2008; 222(6):391–396

[26] Turan-Vural E, Torun-Acar B, Kivanc SA, Acar S. The effect of topical 0.05% cyclosporine on recurrence following pterygium surgery. Clin Ophthalmol. 2011; 5:881–885

[27] Özülken K, Koç M, Ayar O, Hasiripi H. Topical cyclosporine A administration after pterygium surgery. Eur J Ophthalmol. 2012; 22 Suppl 7:S5–S10

[28] Tassman IS. Experimental studies with physiologic glue (autogenous plasma plus thrombin) for use in the eyes. Am J Ophthalmol. 1950; 33(6):870–878

[29] Town AE, Naidoff D. Fibrin closure in eye surgery. Am J Ophthalmol. 1950; 33(6):879–882

[30] Zloto O, Greenbaum E, Fabian ID, Ben Simon GJ. Evicel versus Tisseel versus sutures for attaching conjunctival autograft in pterygium surgery: a prospective comparative clinical study. Ophthalmology. 2017; 124(1):61–65

[31] Romano V, Cruciani M, Conti L, Fontana L. Fibrin glue versus sutures for conjunctival autografting in primary pterygium surgery. Cochrane Database Syst Rev. 2016; 12:CD011308

[32] Maiti R, Mukherjee S, Hota D. Recurrence rate and graft stability with fibrin glue compared with suture and autologous blood coagulum for conjunctival autograft adherence in pterygium surgery: a meta-analysis. Cornea. 2017; 36(10):1285–1294

[33] Alamdari DH, Sedaghat MR, Alizadeh R, Zarei-Ghanavati S, Naseri H, Sharifi F. Comparison of autologous fibrin glue versus nylon sutures for securing conjunctival autografting in pterygium surgery. Int Ophthalmol. 2017

[34] Foroutan A, Beigzadeh F, Ghaempanah MJ, et al. Efficacy of autologous fibrin glue for primary pterygium surgery with conjunctival autograft. Iran J Ophthalmol. 2011; 23(1):39–47

[35] Sati A, Shankar S, Jha A, Kalra D, Mishra S, Gurunadh VS. Comparison of efficacy of three surgical methods of conjunctival autograft fixation in the treatment of pterygium. Int J Ophthalmol. 2014; 34(6):1233–1239

[36] Boucher S, Conlon R, Teja S, et al. Fibrin glue versus autologous blood for conjunctival autograft fixation in pterygium surgery. Can J Ophthalmol. 2015; 50(4):269–272

[37] Bondalapati S, Ambati B. Minimally invasive pterygium surgery: sutureless excision with amniotic membrane and hydrogel sealant. Case Rep Ophthalmol. 2016; 7(1):79–84–. eCollection 2016 Jan-Apr

[38] Xu F, Li M, Yan Y, Lu K, Cui L, Chen Q. A novel technique of sutureless and glueless conjunctival autografting in pterygium surgery by electrocautery pen. Cornea. 2013; 32(3):290–295

[39] Paris FdosS, de Farias CC, Melo GB, Dos Santos MS, Batista JL, Gomes JA. Postoperative subconjunctival corticosteroid injection to prevent pterygium recurrence. Cornea. 2008; 27(4):406–410

[40] Kheirkhah A, Nazari R, Safi H, Ghassemi H, Behrouz MJ, Raju VK. Effects of intraoperative steroid injection on the outcome of pterygium surgery. Eye (Lond). 2013; 27(8):906–914

[41] Prabhasawat P, Tesavibul N, Leelapatranura K, Phonjan T. Efficacy of subconjunctival 5-fluorouracil and triamcinolone injection in impending recurrent pterygium. Ophthalmology. 2006; 113(7):1102–1109

[42] Viani GA, Stefano EJ, De Fendi LI, Fonseca EC. Long-term results and prognostic factors of fractionated strontium-90 eye applicator for pterygium. Int J Radiat Oncol Biol Phys. 2008; 72(4):1174–1179

[43] Qin XJ, Chen HM, Guo L, Guo YY. Low-dose strontium-90 irradiation is effective in preventing the recurrence of pterygia: a ten-year study. PLoS One. 2012; 7(8):e43500

[44] Ali AM, Thariat J, Bensadoun RJ, et al. The role of radiotherapy in the treatment of pterygium: a review of the literature including more than 6000 treated lesions. Cancer Radiother. 2011; 15(2):140–147

[45] MacKenzie FD, Hirst LW, Kynaston B, Bain C. Recurrence rate and complications after beta irradiation for pterygia. Ophthalmology. 1991; 98(12):1776–1780, discussion 1781

10 Nonsurgical Management of Irregular Astigmatism Associated with Pterygium

Melissa Barnett, Thomas P. Arnold, Nathan Schramm, Andrew S. Morgenstern, Christine W. Sindt, and Tracy Schroeder Swartz

Abstract

This chapter describes the role of optometry in the evaluation, care, and management of pterygium patients. When surgical intervention is not indicated, alternative treatment strategies are described. Innovations in scleral lenses such as notching, microvaults, and impression molding are discussed.

Keywords: MD/OD, conjunctival intraepithelial neoplasm (CIN), scleral contact lens, notching, microvault, impression molding, limbus, toric

10.1 Introduction

Pterygia cause irregular astigmatism in increasing amounts as they encroach upon the cornea (▶ Fig. 10.1). According to the Blue Mountains Eye Study of 3,564 people aged 49 years or older, 266 individuals (7.3%) had pterygium (or a history of pterygium surgery) and 2,521 (69.5%) had pinguecula present in either eye.[1] Significantly more men than women had both pinguecula and pterygium. There were significant associations between pterygium and increased pigmentation (skin and hair color), decreased skin sun sensitivity, and sun-related skin damage. In a study that examined the prevalence of pinguecula and pterygium in a general population in Spain of 1,155 people age 40 years and older, the prevalence of pinguecula was 47.9% and increased significantly with age.[2] The prevalence of pterygium was 5.9%; this also increased significantly with age. Of interest, after controlling for age and sex, pinguecula was strongly associated with alcohol intake.[2]

Irregular astigmatism secondary to radial keratotomy, keratoconus, or decentered hyperopic LASIK may be addressed using specialty corneal transplants or topography-guided surface ablation. This is not the case of irregular astigmatism resulting from pterygium, and not all patients may be good candidates for pterygium surgery. They may live too far from a capable surgeon, lack the

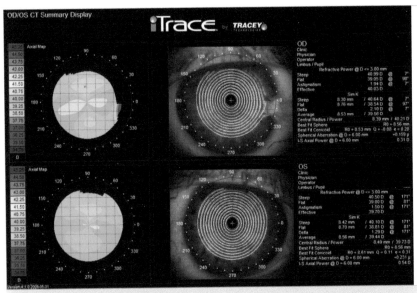

Fig. 10.1 A mild pterygium nasally OD causing more astigmatism than the fellow eye. The axial map demonstrates central astigmatism (bowtie) with a blue island of flattening overlying the lesion (upper left map). The keratometry view demonstrates the lesion nasally.

financial means, or be wary of surgery. The irregular astigmatism must be corrected nonsurgically to allow them to function. Scleral lenses address irregular astigmatism, dry eye disease, visual function, and pain associated with this condition.

Elevated lesions of the conjunctiva such as pingueculae and pterygia[3] often present challenges in fitting the patient desiring refractive correction with contact lenses. These may be a mild pinguecula or conjunctival cyst, more significant, such as in the case of pterygium, (▶ Fig. 10.2 and ▶ Fig. 10.3) or status post trabeculectomy, shunt, stent, or glaucoma implant. Intraocular pressure may be compromised if there is excessive pressure or rubbing over tube shunts or valves. This may lead to conjunctival or tube erosion, increasing the risk of further complications such as endophthalmitis. Elevations on surface of the cornea such as in Salzmann's nodular degeneration (▶ Fig. 10.4) or severe corneal scarring also complicate lens fitting.

Another indication for scleral lens fitting is control of ocular surface disease (OSD).[4] Unlike conventional contact lenses, scleral lenses vault the cornea, and land on the scleral conjunctiva. The fluid reservoir continuously bathes and hydrates the cornea. The lens serves as a barrier to protect the corneal and conjunctival surface while blinking. Scleral lenses have also been reported to reduce inflammatory mediators, which may cause pterygium progression. La Porta Weber et al studied osmolarity in a group of 25 patients with OSD. A decrease in tear film osmolarity after 12 months of scleral lens wear was reported.[5] Carracedo and colleagues found statistically significant decreases in tear osmolarity and diadenosine tetraphosphate after patients wore scleral lenses for 6 to 9 hours.[6] Scleral lenses have been found to be beneficial n multiple conditions including ocular surface disease, vernal keratoconjuncitivits,[7] advanced atopic keratoconjuctivitis,[8] graft versus host disease,[9,10] neurotrophic keratitis, graft versus

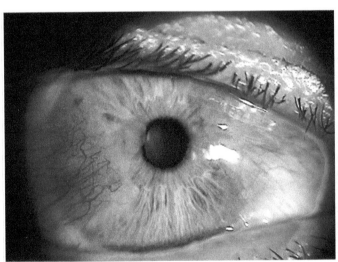

Fig. 10.2 Larger pterygia located both nasally and temporally.

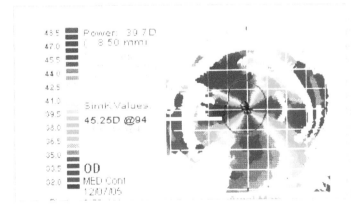

Fig. 10.3 Topography map corresponding to the ▶ Fig. 10.2. Note the appearance of two bowties 90 degrees apart.

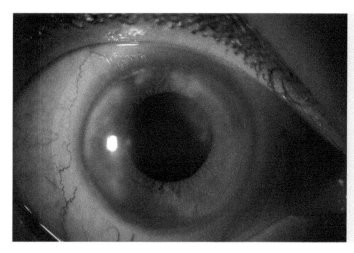

Fig. 10.4 Corneal elevations in Salzmann's nodular degeneration.

host disease, Steven Johnsons Syndrome, ocular cicatricial pemphigoid, limbal stem cell deficiency amongst others. Scleral lenses do not appear to reduce matrix metalloproteinases, however.[6] Periodic visits for these patients are required to maintain adequate control of OSD, reduce risk of progression, and avoid surgery.

With the increased interest in scleral lenses as a desirable alternative in fitting the irregular cornea or conjunctiva with elevated lesions, new strategies are required and new technologies developed. Corneal topography or Scheimpflug tomography is typically used to assess corneal curvature in corneal gas permeable fitting but is less useful for scleral lens fitting as data is not collected for the limbus or sclera. Anterior segment optical coherence tomography (OCT) is now commonly employed in scleral lens fitting. OCT can be used to measure lens thickness centrally and peripherally, examine lens edges for flaws and causes of discomfort, measure posterior tear film thickness, and assess points of lens bearing to determine the need for design modification.[11] Anterior OCT software contains linear calipers to allow precise analysis of the anterior segment at various sagittal depths. Angular calipers allow measurement of corneal, limbal, and scleral angles to assist in fitting.[11]

10.2 Fitting Strategies

Various fitting strategies are used to fit lenses in these complicated patients. Simply ordering lens specifications such as optic zone radius, total diameter, back vertex power, and material is not adequate in complicated eyes. Custom specifications including tertiary and secondary curvatures, asphericity, diameter, and optic zone modifications are often required. For simplicity, customization can be categorized in three areas: the optical zone, the transition zone, and the landing zone. Unlike regular corneal gas permeable lenses with back surface powers in alignment with the corneal surface, scleral lenses have a post lens tear reservoir between the posterior lens surface and anterior cornea. The transition zone is located just peripheral to the optical zone chord continuing to the beginning of the presumed or measured landing zone chord. It varies with each manufacturer and design. It has been previously referred to as the limbal or intermediate zone. It is described by its radius of curvature and its width.

The landing zone is located peripheral to the transitional zone and begins from the primary functional diameter and ends at the lens edge. It may also be a planar (flat) surface placed at various angles from the transitional zone to the edge of the lens. Also described as lens haptics. It is described by its radius of curvature and its width.

These zones can be customized to maintain good functional vision and minimal discomfort despite elevated lisions. Techniques specific to fitting patients with pterygium and conjunctival elevations include adjusting the lens diameter, notching the lens, and custom vaulting techniques.

A standard corneal gas permeable lens diameter of 9.0 to 9.5 mm may encounter the elevated lesion, and prolonged contact may cause irritation, inflammation and discomfort. If the lesions are encroaching significantly onto the cornea, it is possible to fit a gas permeable lens inside the lesion's borders by decreasing the lens diameter. If the lesion is a pinguecula 2 to 3 mm beyond the limbus, a proven strategy of fitting a smaller diameter lens may be the most straightforward solution.

Table 10.1 Scleral lens categories

	Lens diameters (mm)
Corneo-scleral	12.9–13.5
Semi-scleral	13.6–14.9
Mini-scleral	15.0–18.0
Full scleral	18.1–24.0 or greater

Source: Reproduced with permission of Contact Lens Spectrum, published October 2010. Contact Lens Spectrum is published monthly by PentaVision LLC, ©2010 All rights reserved. Visit www.clspectrum.com for more information.

This works well in eyes with a relatively small horizontal visible iris diameter. This has been defined as a diameter of 11.5 mm or less.[2] Alternatively, if the elevation is located at the limbus, increasing the diameter to vault the elevation may be more successful. Scleral lens fitting categories and diameters are described in ▶ Table 10.1.

In patients with peripheral corneal or conjunctival lesions, evaluation of peripheral fitting characteristics is essential. Conjunctival blanching and impingement must be avoided in these patients.[12] Blanching is a whitening of the conjunctiva due to lens pressure on the tissue. Changing the peripheral curves or using a nonrotationally symmetrical lens may alleviate blanching.[13] Impingement occurs when the edge of the lens focally pinches into the conjunctival tissue. Impingement can occur as a result of a very steep landing zone with minimal contact with the conjunctiva except for the very edge of the lens. Conjunctival staining and hypertrophy may be evident after lens removal. To alleviate impingement, flatten the scleral landing zone periphery or increase the edge lift. It is also possible to increase the overall diameter of the lens to bear the weight more evenly on the conjunctival surface.

For a large irregular elevation, it is possible to at the edge of the scleral lens to avoid direct contact. The patient is instructed to align the lens notch is a specific position to avoid the conjunctival elevation. The notch itself helps to keep the lens situated. Additionally, however, toric peripheral curves of at least 150-μm difference may be employed[2] (▶ Fig. 10.4). The first step is to measure the length and width of the conjunctival abnormality with a slit beam of the biomicroscope or using scleral topography/profilometry. The height and width of the conjunctival abnormality with the scleral lens on the eye are then measured. The scleral lens is marked with a sharpie or dry erase marker with the lens on the eye. Be sure to inform the patient that the lens is being marked and not the eye. Finally, measure the marking on the lens after the scleral lens is removed. Consult the preferred laboratory consultant to discuss the notch and send the measurements and/or the lens to the laboratory. Notching is performed manually and is not precisely reproducible.

When inserting the scleral lens with a notch, it is important to place it on the eye with the correct orientation. Be sure to inform the staff person who is training the patient on scleral lens application and removal, as well as the patient, about the need for proper lens orientation.

Pterygia and Salzmann's nodular dystrophy can be even more complex as they involve the cornea itself. Irregular astigmatism may reduce vision. A unique and successful solution involves a "microvault." This is a raised dome either on the edge or within the body of the scleral lens (▶ Fig. 10.5). The practitioner describes to the laboratory consultant the exact location and desired height of the vault. The following must be specified[14]:

- The axis—"the optical axis location of the center of the microvault relative to the center of the lens and whether the microvault is nasal or temporal."
- The amount of decentration—"distance from the center of the lens to the center of the microvault."
- The width—"equal to the width of the microvault."
- The depth—"the sagittal depth of the microvault: how high the apex of the vault is above the ocular surface (up to 500 μm)."[6]

Another option offered by some manufacturers is a focal vaulting feature located at the edge or within the lens (▶ Fig. 10.6). A spherical elevation is created centrally within the lens, and a hemispherical ripple is created at the lens landing zone, while maintaining the circular shape of the lens edge. The focal feature vaults over a peripheral corneal or conjunctival elevation. First, the axis of the elevation relative to the center of the lens is noted. Its distance from the center of the lens is determined by measuring the extent of the elevation from the edge. Finally, the width and depth of the central or peripheral vault feature is quantified.

Alternatively, a hybrid, gas permeable lens, may be used. The soft skirt of a hybrid lens drapes over the peripheral elevation.

An advanced design with custom, impression-based scleral lens technology such as an EyePrint-Pro (EyePrint Prosthetics, Denver, CO) may be

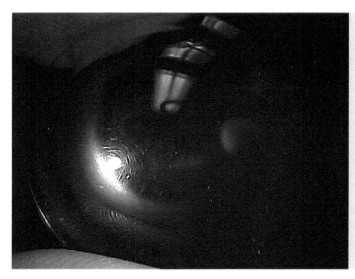

Fig. 10.5 Image of focal vault within the lens.

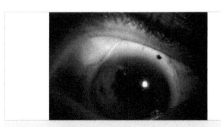

Fig. 10.6 Image of scleral lens notch.

used. An impression of the ocular surface is created, and sent to the lab for digitizing and design of the custom prosthetic scleral cover shell. Three-dimensional scanning and computer numerically controlled machining systems create an exact match to the irregular ocular surface.[15] The prosthetic scleral cover shell may also be used to avoid pressure on the conjunctiva and contact with the surgical area.

It is important to remember nonsurgical alternatives for correction in patients with pterygia and other ocular elevations. While these techniques are complicated, they are highly successful in creating functional vision correction with good comfort in patients who are unable or unwilling to pursue surgery. Scleral lenses may also control OSD and minimize risk of progression.

References

[1] Panchapakesan J, Hourihan F, Mitchell P. Prevalence of pterygium and pinguecula: the Blue Mountains Eye Study. Aust N Z J Ophthalmol. 1998; 26 Suppl 1:S2–S5

[2] Caroline PJ, Andre MP. Elevated conjunctival lesions and scleral lenses. Contact Lens Spectr. 2017; 32(February):56

[3] Bennett ES, Weissman BA. Clinical Contact Lens Practice. Philadelphia, PA: Lippincott, Williams & Wilkins; 2005:198

[4] Schornack MM, Pyle J, Patel SV. Scleral lenses in the management of ocular surface disease. Ophthalmology. 2014; 121 (7):1398–1405

[5] La Porta Weber S, Becco de Souza R, Gomes JÁP, Hofling-Lima AL. The use of the esclera scleral contact lens in the treatment of moderate to severe dry eye disease. Am J Ophthalmol. 2016; 163:167–173.e1

[6] Carracedo G, Blanco MS, Martin-Gil A, Zicheng W, Alvarez JC, Pintor J. Short-term effect of scleral lens on the dry eye biomarkers in keratoconus. Optom Vis Sci. 2016; 93(2):150–157

[7] Rathi VM, Sudharman Mandathara P, Vaddavalli PK, Dumpati S, Chakrabarti T, Sangwan VS. Fluid-filled scleral contact lenses in vernal keratoconjunctivitis. Eye Contact Lens. 2012; 38(3):203–206

[8] Margolis R, Thakrar V, Perez VL. Role of rigid gas-permeable scleral contact lenses in the management of advanced atopic keratoconjunctivitis. Cornea. 2007; 26(9):1032–1034

[9] Kim SK. Update on ocular graft versus host disease. Curr Opin Ophthalmol. 2006; 17(4):344–348

[10] Kim SK. Ocular graft vs. host disease. Ocul Surf. 2005; 3(4) Suppl:S177–S179

[11] Kojima R, Caroline P, Walker M, Kinoshita B, André M, Lampa M. Benefits of OCT when fitting specialty lenses: anterior segment optical coherence tomography can be used for many pre- and post-contact lens assessments. Contact Lens Spectr. 2014; 29(October):1

[12] M Barnett. 10 Tips for Smarter Scleral Lens Fitting. Review of Cornea and Contact Lenses, Review of Optometry. October 15, 2012. Available at: http:/reviewofcontactlenses.com/content/c/37103/. Accessed October 15, 2017

[13] Barnett M, Johns LK. Contemporary Scleral Lenses: Theory and Application, Volume 4. Sharjah: Bentham Science Publishers; 2017

[14] Zenlens MicroVault. Bausch & Lomb Specialty Vision Products. Available at: www.aldenoptical.com.Zenlens_Micro-Vault_Promo.pdf

[15] The Science Behind EyePrintPRO™. Available at: https://www.eyeprintpro.com/our-science/. Accessed October 15, 2017

11 Stem Cell Applications in Pterygium

Abhinav Loomba and Virender Singh Sangwan

Abstract

In this chapter, we describe briefly the pathophysiology of pterygium and how stem cell deficiency results in pterygium. We review how to identify limbal stem cells and their role in pterygium. Novel surgical technique of stem cell transplant in pterygium surgery is discussed.

Keywords: pterygium, stem cell deficiency, stem cells, pterygium surgery, SLET, limbal stem cells

11.1 Introduction

Pterygium is a benign, wing-shaped fibrovascular proliferation extending onto the cornea. As of today, there are many approaches to its treatment once it is decided that surgical intervention is required. The most common surgical techniques include excision of pterygium with bare sclera, using a conjunctival or conjunctival limbal autograft, coverage with amniotic membrane (AM), or the use of adjuncts such as mitomycin C. Recurrence rates among these techniques vary widely, with reports as high as 88% for the bare sclera technique[1,2,3] and more comparable results among the other mentioned techniques, with a recurrence rate between 0.003 and 40.9%. Conjunctival-limbal autograft offers a low recurrence rate and fewer complications.[4,5,6,7]

The major environmental factor for pterygium generation is exposure to ultraviolet (UV) light. Therefore, pterygium has a worldwide distribution and common in peri-equatorial latitudes 37° north and south of the equator, forming a so-called pterygium belt.

Some advantages of using an AM are inhibition of angiogenesis and the possibility to cover a large area without the need of harvesting healthy conjunctiva. Nevertheless, the cosmetic results, postoperative inflammation, and recurrence rates are higher with AM transplantation than they are with conjunctival limbal autografts.[8,9,10]

11.2 Pathophysiology

UV radiation (UVR) is damaging for the eye, resulting in a reduction or even loss of vision. The cornea is particularly susceptible to UVR due to its natural transparency and its shape, which contributes to a peripheral light focusing effect, affecting the nasal limbus where UV irradiation is 20-fold stronger.[11,12] This is the most frequent site for the onset of pterygium, a noncancerous growth of the cornea, usually bilateral, which occupies the corneal equator. The pterygium disrupts the limbal barrier, which separates the cornea from the conjunctiva and centripetally invades the cornea surface. It is characterized by squamous hyperplasia and goblet cell hyperplasia. In advanced cases, the visual axis may be covered by vascularized opaque tissue, thus leading to discomfort, deterioration of vision, or even blindness[13] As such dramatic phenotype changes occur in the limbus and its adjacent tissues, alterations in the limbal stem cell niche and its resident limbal epithelial stem cells (LESCs) must also occur. LESCs play a key role in the maintenance of cornea transparency and homeostasis by replenishing its outermost layer, the epithelium.[14] If these stem cells become depleted by injury or disease, the neighboring conjunctival epithelium infringes onto the corneal surface causing vascularization, persistent epithelial breakdown, severe pain, and blindness[15] Although an LESC specific marker remains elusive, the expression of certain proteins, including P63α, ABCG2, and cytokeratin 15 and more recently ABCB5,[16] has been recognized as putative stem cell markers for these cells.[15] High levels of putative stem cell marker expression combined with high colony-forming efficiency[17] are indicative of the stem cell phenotype.

11.2.1 Stem Cells

The major role of cell division in adult life is to maintain the number of differentiated cells at a constant level, that is, to replace cells that have died or been lost through injury. The rate at which new cells are produced is a measure of how rapidly the cell population is turning over. Tissues with a permanently renewing cell population, such as blood, testis, and stratified squamous epithelia (including corneal epithelium), are characterized by rapid and continuous cell turnover; the terminally differentiated cells have a short life span and are replaced through proliferation of a distinct subpopulation of cells, known as stem cells.[18,19] Stem cells are a small subpopulation of the total tissue. Potten and Loeffler[20,21,22] defined stem cells, by virtue of their functional attributes, as "undifferentiated cells capable of

- Proliferation.
- Self-maintenance.
- Producing a large number of differentiated, functional progeny.
- Regenerating the tissue after injury.
- A flexibility in the use of these options.

11.2.2 Characteristics of Stem Cells

- Stem cells are poorly differentiated; the cytoplasm of stem cells appears primitive and contains few, if any, differentiation products.
- Stem cells have a high capacity for self-renewal, with an increased potential for error-free proliferation and cell division. Error-free proliferation is essential, as any genetic error at the level of stem cells will continuously and permanently pass on to the whole clone of cells, resulting in abnormal differentiation and cellular dysfunction.
- Stem cells have a long life span, which might be equivalent to the life of the organism in which they reside.
- Stem cells have a long cell cycle time or slow cycling (which indicates low mitotic activity). Although stem cells are endowed with high proliferative potential, under steady-state conditions they exhibit extremely low rates of proliferation.
- Cell division within stem cells can be intrinsically asymmetric, asymmetric only with regard to daughter cell fate, or symmetric. When cell division is obligatorily asymmetric, one of the daughter cells remains as its parent and serves to replenish the stem cell pool, whereas the other daughter cell is destined to divide and differentiate with the acquisition of features that characterize the specific tissue. On the other hand, the asymmetry in division may be determined by the local environment, which induces otherwise similar daughter cells to behave differently.
- Finally, all divisions of the stem cell may be symmetric, but are "self-renewing" only half the time.

Regardless of which mechanism is operative during or soon after cell division, one of the daughter cells may follow the path of differentiation. Such a cell is called a "transient amplifying cell" and is less primitive than its parent stem cell. Transient amplifying cells divide more frequently than stem cells, but have a limited proliferative potential and are considered the initial step of a pathway that results in terminal differentiation. They differentiate into "postmitotic cells" and, finally, to "terminally differentiated cells." Both postmitotic and terminally differentiated cells are incapable of cell division.

Stem cells are usually under protection. In the hemopoietic system, stem cells are stored in bone marrow; in all epithelial tissues, stem cells are in the basal layer. In the corneal epithelium, the stem cells are located in the basal layer at the limbus.[23]

11.2.3 Identification of Limbal Stem Cells

The concept that epithelial cells in the limbal region are involved in the renewal of corneal epithelium was first proposed by Davanger and Evensen in 1971.[24] In healed eccentric corneal epithelial defects in heavily pigmented eyes, they observed pigmented epithelial migration lines (cells) that migrated from the limbal region toward the central cornea.[24] They suggested that the limbal papillary structure (palisades of Vogt) serves as a generative organ for corneal epithelial cells. Later, experimental studies by Schermer et al[25] and Cotsarelis et al[26] confirmed that the source of cell proliferation and migration after a corneal epithelial defect is the sclerocorneal limbus.

- The limbal basal epithelium contains the least differentiated cells of the corneal epithelium. Epithelial cells contain different types of keratins, some of which indicate a high level of differentiation, whereas others are found mostly in less differentiated cells.[25,27,28]

The differential expression of keratins allows the separation of cell populations within the corneal epithelium according to their level of differentiation, though no markers have yet been identified to label LESCs. The 64 KD keratin K3 indicates a cornea-specific type of differentiation. It was observed that keratin K3 exists in the suprabasal epithelium of the limbus and the entire corneal epithelium, but is not expressed in either the limbal basal epithelium or the adjacent bulbar conjunctiva.[25] This observation led to the hypothesis that the limbal basal epithelium lacks a differentiated cornea-type phenotype, and therefore contains the least differentiated cells of the epithelium (i.e., stem cells). The limbal basal epithelium also lacks the expression of the corneal-specific keratin K12, which is expressed in both the suprabasal limbal epithelium and the entire corneal epithelium.[29]

- The limbal basal epithelium contains cells that exhibit the proliferative characteristics of stem cells. Limbal basal epithelial cells have a higher proliferative potential in culture than central and peripheral corneal epithelial cells.[30,31] Limbal basal cells respond to central corneal wounds and to tumor-promoting agents by undergoing higher proliferation than central corneal epithelial cells, which terminate proliferation-initiating differentiation.[26]

Labeling studies have demonstrated that the mitotic index of the corneal epithelium tends to be higher toward the periphery, suggesting that the peripheral corneal basal cells are more active in DNA synthesis.[32]

- Further support for the limbal location of corneal epithelial stem cells is derived from experimental studies and clinical observations of abnormal corneal epithelial wound healing when the limbal epithelium is partially or completely removed. These studies produced a spectrum of corneal surface abnormalities characterized by conjunctival epithelial ingrowth (conjunctivalization), vascularization, and chronic inflammation, which indicated limbal stem cell deficiency. The conjunctival source of the epithelial ingrowth was proved by immunofluorescent staining with monoclonal antibodies and by the detection of goblet cells with impression cytology.[33,34,35,36]

11.2.4 Different Surgical Techniques in Pterygium Excision

With time, different techniques have been employed for the excision of pterygium. One of the first techniques was simple excision with bare sclera. The reported rate of recurrence after simple excision without adjuvant treatment ranges from 24 to 89%.[37] Several techniques have been developed to reduce the recurrence rate, including limbal conjunctival autograft,[38] intraoperative or postoperative application of mitomycin C,[39] bulbar conjunctival autograft,[40] AM transplantation,[41] radiation,[42] photodynamic therapy,[43] antiangiogenic agents,[44] and the combination of two or more of these methods.[45]

11.2.5 Role of Conjunctival Autograft in Surgical Management of Pterygium

The procedure involves obtaining an autograft, usually from the superotemporal bulbar conjunctiva, and suturing the graft over the exposed scleral bed after excision of the pterygium. The graft can be either sutured or secured with fibrin glue. Stark and coworkers[46] stress the importance of careful dissection of Tenon's tissue from the conjunctival graft and recipient bed, minimal manipulation of tissue, and accurate orientation of the graft. Lawrence W. Hirst, MBBS, from Australia recommends using a large incision for pterygium excision and a large graft and has reported a very low recurrence rate with this technique.[47]

Conjunctival or limbal conjunctival autografts are suggested to be the best treatment with a low recurrence rate ranging from 1.9 to 5.3%, and high safety according to some studies.[48,49,50,51] Furthermore, they have been demonstrated to be more effective at treating recurrent pterygium than other methods.[52]

A meta-analysis to further explore the association between the application of fibrin glue in pterygium surgery and the recurrence rate, complication rate, and surgical duration was conducted. In total, 1,839 eyes from 24 studies were included in the meta-analysis. Based on the overall meta-analysis, it was found that, compared with sutures, fibrin glue was more effective at reducing the recurrence rate, but not the complication rate. Analysis indicated a significantly shorter surgical duration for fibrin glue compared with sutures. In the subgroup analysis, based on region, follow-up time, quality score, sample size, study type, and suture material, fibrin glue still had a lower recurrence rate. Moreover, there were no significant differences in complication rates between the two groups in terms of region, sample size, study type, and suture material.[53]

11.2.6 Mini-SLET for Pterygium Treatment

Conjunctival-limbal autograft offers a low recurrence rate and fewer complications; however, it cannot be performed in cases where a large defect needs to be covered or in patients where the conjunctiva needs to be preserved for future glaucoma surgery to avoid conjunctival scarring at the harvesting site.

A novel technique has been described by Hernández-Bogantes et al,[54] taking advantage of the properties of AM and LESCs. This technique describes the use of an AM graft to cover the bare sclera area combined with a small autologous simple limbal epithelial transplant (mini-SLET) to provide stem cells at the limbal area.

A total of 10 eyes underwent pterygium excision with AM coverage of the bare sclera and placement of pieces of limbal epithelium in a linear fashion in the affected limbal area covered by a second AM using fibrin glue. After up to 8 months of follow-up, there were no signs of early recurrence or sight-threatening complications. The minor ipsilateral simple limbal epithelial transplantation technique for the treatment of pterygium requires less tissue than the conventional conjunctival autograft, leaving healthy conjunctiva if needed for another procedure in the future, and offers the advantages of epithelial stem cells, which in the long term may reduce the rate of recurrence significantly.[54]

11.2.7 Surgical Technique and Steps of SLET in Pterygium Excision Surgery

- Parts of the eye are painted with betadine and draped maintaining sterility (▶ Fig. 11.1).
- Using a Lim's forceps, the body of pterygium is grasped and subconjunctival dissection done with Vannas scissors from forniceal approach (▶ Fig. 11.2).

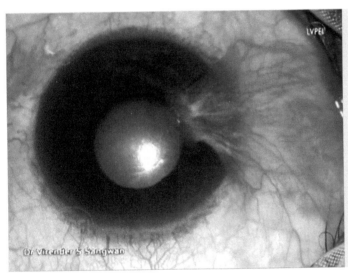

Fig. 11.1 Grade III pterygium: parts of the eye are painted with betadine and draped maintaining sterility.

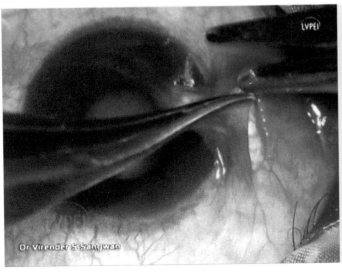

Fig. 11.2 Using a Lim's forceps, the body of pterygium is grasped and subconjunctival dissection done with Vannas scissors from forniceal approach.

- Once the plane is identified, the head of the pterygium is separated and peeled off using forceps and the conjunctiva falls back toward the fornix (▶ Fig. 11.3 and ▶ Fig. 11.4).
- Snip biopsy of the limbus with stem cells is taken using Vannas and chopped into three to four pieces (▶ Fig. 11.5, ▶ Fig. 11.6, ▶ Fig. 11.7).
- Pieces are placed over the limbus and the bare sclera, and secured using fibrin and thrombin glue (▶ Fig. 11.8).

- After the glue settles (1–2 minutes), bandage contact lens is placed over the cornea.
- Betadine eye drops are instilled and eye patched.
- Postoperative management consists of removing the patch next day and using topical steroids in tapering fashion for 8 to 12 weeks and topical antibiotics for 1 to 2 weeks or until surface epithelium heals and no epithelial defect observed.

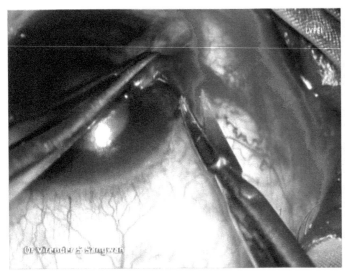

Fig. 11.3 Once the plane is identified, the head of the pterygium is separated and peeled off using forceps and Vannas scissors.

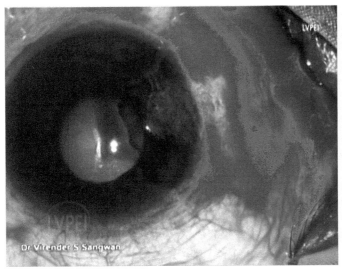

Fig. 11.4 After the pterygium is separated and peeled off, the conjunctiva falls back toward the fornix.

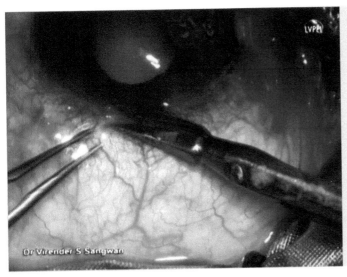

Fig. 11.5 Landmark for snip biopsy for stem cells to be taken near the limbus.

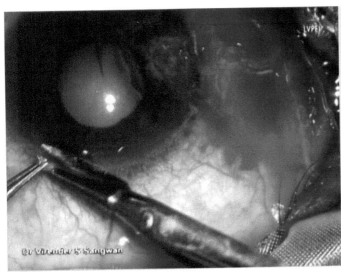

Fig. 11.6 Snip biopsy of the limbus with stem cells is taken using Lim's forceps and cut with Vannas.

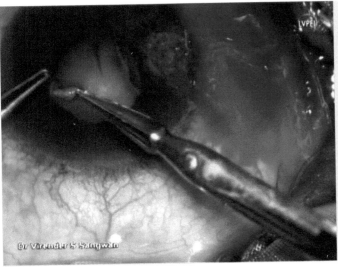

Fig. 11.7 Snip biopsy of the limbus with stem cells is chopped into three to four pieces using Vannas.

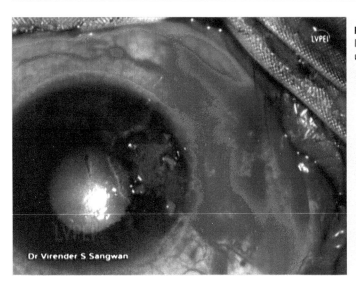

Fig. 11.8 Pieces are placed over the limbus and the bare sclera and secured using fibrin and thrombin glue.

References

[1] Cano-Parra J, Diaz-Llopis M, Maldonado MJ, Vila E, Menezo JL. Prospective trial of intraoperative mitomycin C in the treatment of primary pterygium. Br J Ophthalmol. 1995; 79 (5):439–441

[2] Demirok A, Simsek S, Cinal A, Yasar T. Intraoperative application of mitomycin C in the surgical treatment of pterygium. Eur J Ophthalmol. 1998; 8(3):153–156

[3] Ozer A, Yildirim N, Erol N, Yurdakul S. Long-term results of bare sclera, limbal-conjunctival autograft and amniotic membrane graft techniques in primary pterygium excisions. Ophthalmologica. 2009; 223(4):269–273

[4] Hirst LW. Recurrence and complications after 1,000 surgeries using pterygium extended removal followed by extended conjunctival transplant. Ophthalmology. 2012; 119(11): 2205–2210

[5] Chen PP, Ariyasu RG, Kaza V, LaBree LD, McDonnell PJ. A randomized trial comparing mitomycin C and conjunctival autograft after excision of primary pterygium. Am J Ophthalmol. 1995; 120(2):151–160

[6] Tananuvat N, Martin T. The results of amniotic membrane transplantation for primary pterygium compared with conjunctival autograft. Cornea. 2004; 23(5):458–463

[7] Malek I, Zghal I, Chebbi A, et al. Conjunctival limbal autograft versus simple excision with intra-operative mitomycin C in pterygium surgery: a comparative study [in French]. J Fr Ophtalmol. 2013; 36(3):230–235

[8] Kenyon KR. Amniotic membrane: mother's own remedy for ocular surface disease. Cornea. 2005; 24(6):639–642

[9] Li M, Zhu M, Yu Y, Gong L, Zhao N, Robitaille MJ. Comparison of conjunctival autograft transplantation and amniotic membrane transplantation for pterygium: a meta-analysis. Graefes Arch Clin Exp Ophthalmol. 2012; 250(3):375–381

[10] Kheirkhah A, Nazari R, Nikdel M, Ghassemi H, Hashemi H, Behrouz MJ. Postoperative conjunctival inflammation after pterygium surgery with amniotic membrane transplantation versus conjunctival autograft. Am J Ophthalmol. 2011; 152 (5):733–738

[11] Coroneo MT, Müller-Stolzenburg NW, Ho A. Peripheral light focusing by the anterior eye and the ophthalmohelioses. Ophthalmic Surg. 1991; 22(12):705–711

[12] Maloof AJ, Ho A, Coroneo MT. Influence of corneal shape on limbal light focusing. Invest Ophthalmol Vis Sci. 1994; 35(5): 2592–2598

[13] Bradley JC, Yang W, Bradley RH, Reid TW, Schwab IR. The science of pterygia. Br J Ophthalmol. 2010; 94(7):815–820

[14] Notara M, Alatza A, Gilfillan J, et al. In sickness and in health: Corneal epithelial stem cell biology, pathology and therapy. Exp Eye Res. 2010; 90(2):188–195

[15] Notara M, Daniels JT. Biological principals and clinical potentials of limbal epithelial stem cells. Cell Tissue Res. 2008; 331 (1):135–143

[16] Ksander BR, Kolovou PE, Wilson BJ, et al. ABCB5 is a limbal stem cell gene required for corneal development and repair. Nature. 2014; 511(7509):353–357

[17] Barrandon Y, Green H. Three clonal types of keratinocyte with different capacities for multiplication. Proc Natl Acad Sci U S A. 1987; 84(8):2302–2306

[18] Hall PA, Watt FM. Stem cells: the generation and maintenance of cellular diversity. Development. 1989; 106(4):619–633

[19] Miller SJ, Lavker RM, Sun TT. Keratinocyte stem cells of cornea, skin, and hair follicle: common and distinguishing features. Semin Dev Biol. 1993; 4(4):217–240

[20] Potten CS, Loeffler M. Stem cells: attributes, cycles, spirals, pitfalls and uncertainties. Lessons for and from the crypt. Development. 1990; 110(4):1001–1020

[21] Potten CS, Morris RJ. Epithelial stem cells in vivo. J Cell Sci Suppl. 1988; 10 Suppl:45–62

[22] Potten SC, Loeffler M. Epidermal cell proliferation. I. Changes with time in the proportion of isolated, paired and clustered labeled cells in sheets of murine epidermis. Virchows Arch. 1987; 53:286–300

[23] Dua HS, Azuara-Blanco A. Limbal stem cells of the corneal epithelium. Surv Ophthalmol. 2000; 44(5):415–425

[24] Davanger M, Evensen A. Role of the pericorneal papillary structure in renewal of corneal epithelium. Nature. 1971; 229(5286):560–561

[25] Schermer A, Galvin S, Sun TT. Differentiation-related expression of a major 64K corneal keratin in vivo and in culture suggests limbal location of corneal epithelial stem cells. J Cell Biol. 1986; 103(1):49–62

[26] Cotsarelis G, Cheng SZ, Dong G, Sun TT, Lavker RM. Existence of slow-cycling limbal epithelial basal cells that can be preferentially stimulated to proliferate: implications on epithelial stem cells. Cell. 1989; 57(2):201–209

[27] Cooper D, Schermer A, Sun TT. Classification of human epithelia and their neoplasms using monoclonal antibodies to keratins: strategies, applications, and limitations. Lab Invest. 1985; 52(3):243–256

[28] Moll R, Franke WW, Schiller DL, Geiger B, Krepler R. The catalog of human cytokeratins: patterns of expression in normal epithelia, tumors and cultured cells. Cell. 1982; 31(1):11–24

[29] Kurpakus MA, Stock EL, Jones JC. Expression of the 55-kD/64-kD corneal keratins in ocular surface epithelium. Invest Ophthalmol Vis Sci. 1990; 31(3):448–456

[30] Ebato B, Friend J, Thoft RA. Comparison of limbal and peripheral human corneal epithelium in tissue culture. Invest Ophthalmol Vis Sci. 1988; 29(10):1533–1537

[31] Lindberg K, Brown ME, Chaves HV, Kenyon KR, Rheinwald JG. In vitro propagation of human ocular surface epithelial cells for transplantation. Invest Ophthalmol Vis Sci. 1993; 34(9):2672–2679

[32] Hanna C, O'Brien JE. Cell production and migration in the epithelial layer of the cornea. Arch Ophthalmol. 1960; 64:536–539

[33] Chen JJ, Tseng SC. Abnormal corneal epithelial wound healing in partial-thickness removal of limbal epithelium. Invest Ophthalmol Vis Sci. 1991; 32(8):2219–2233

[34] Chen JJ, Tseng SC. Corneal epithelial wound healing in partial limbal deficiency. Invest Ophthalmol Vis Sci. 1990; 31(7):1301–1314

[35] Huang AJ, Tseng SC. Corneal epithelial wound healing in the absence of limbal epithelium. Invest Ophthalmol Vis Sci. 1991; 32(1):96–105

[36] Kruse FE, Chen JJ, Tsai RJ, Tseng SC. Conjunctival transdifferentiation is due to the incomplete removal of limbal basal epithelium. Invest Ophthalmol Vis Sci. 1990; 31(9):1903–1913

[37] Jaros PA, DeLuise VP. Pingueculae and pterygia. Surv Ophthalmol. 1988; 33(1):41–49

[38] Basti S, Rao SK. Current status of limbal conjunctival autograft. Curr Opin Ophthalmol. 2000; 11(4):224–232

[39] Pérez-Rico C, Benítez-Herreros J, Montes-Mollón MA, et al. Intraoperative mitomycin C and corneal endothelium after pterygium surgery. Cornea. 2009; 28(10):1135–1138

[40] Nieuwendaal CP, van der Meulen IJ, Mourits M, Lapid-Gortzak R. Long-term follow-up of pterygium surgery using a conjunctival autograft and Tissucol. Cornea. 2011; 30(1):34–36

[41] Jain AK, Bansal R, Sukhija J. Human amniotic membrane transplantation with fibrin glue in management of primary pterygia: a new tuck-in technique. Cornea. 2008; 27(1):94–99

[42] Viani GA, Stefano EJ, De Fendi LI, Fonseca EC. Long-term results and prognostic factors of fractionated strontium-90 eye applicator for pterygium. Int J Radiat Oncol Biol Phys. 2008; 72(4):1174–1179

[43] Fossarello M, Peiretti E, Zucca I, Perra MT, Serra A. Photodynamic therapy of pterygium with verteporfin: a preliminary report. Cornea. 2004; 23(4):330–338

[44] Razeghinejad MR, Hosseini H, Ahmadi F, Rahat F, Eghbal H. Preliminary results of subconjunctival bevacizumab in primary pterygium excision. Ophthalmic Res. 2010; 43(3):134–138

[45] Frucht-Pery J, Raiskup F, Ilsar M, Landau D, Orucov F, Solomon A. Conjunctival autografting combined with low-dose mitomycin C for prevention of primary pterygium recurrence. Am J Ophthalmol. 2006; 141(6):1044–1050

[46] Starck T, Kenyon KR, Serrano F. Conjunctival autograft for primary and recurrent pterygium: surgical technique and problem management. Cornea. 1991; 10(3):196–202

[47] Hirst LW. Prospective study of primary pterygium surgery using pterygium extended removal followed by extended conjunctival transplantation. Ophthalmology. 2008; 115(10):1663–1672

[48] Kenyon KR, Wagoner MD, Hettinger ME. Conjunctival autograft transplantation for advanced and recurrent pterygium. Ophthalmology. 1985; 92(11):1461–1470

[49] Prabhasawat P, Barton K, Burkett G, Tseng SC. Comparison of conjunctival autografts, amniotic membrane grafts, and primary closure for pterygium excision. Ophthalmology. 1997; 104(6):974–985

[50] Sánchez-Thorin JC, Rocha G, Yelin JB. Meta-analysis on the recurrence rates after bare sclera resection with and without mitomycin C use and conjunctival autograft placement in surgery for primary pterygium. Br J Ophthalmol. 1998; 82(6):661–665

[51] Young AL, Leung GY, Wong AK, Cheng LL, Lam DS. A randomised trial comparing 0.02% mitomycin C and limbal conjunctival autograft after excision of primary pterygium. Br J Ophthalmol. 2004; 88(8):995–997

[52] Al Fayez MF. Limbal versus conjunctival autograft transplantation for advanced and recurrent pterygium. Ophthalmology. 2002; 109(9):1752–1755

[53] Lan A, Xiao F, Wang Y, Luo Z, Cao Q. Efficacy of fibrin glue versus sutures for attaching conjunctival autografts in pterygium surgery: a systematic review with meta-analysis and trial sequential analysis of evidence. Oncotarget. 2017; 8(25):41487–41497

[54] Hernández-Bogantes E, Amescua G, Navas A, et al. Minor ipsilateral simple limbal epithelial transplantation (mini-SLET) for pterygium treatment. Br J Ophthalmol. 2015; 99(12):1598–1600

12 Surgical Approach to Isolated and Associated Presentations of Pterygium

Alan N. Carlson

Abstract

Pterygium surgery provides an overview of this ocular finding that is commonly encountered clinically in isolation or in association with other ocular problems, particularly those impacting the cornea and ocular surface. Analysis of various pathways and underlying conditions that are associated and lead to the development of pterygia provides for greater understanding, enhanced patient education, and a more strategic approach that ideally brings about improved long-term success and a decreased recurrence rate.

Keywords: pterygium, ocular rosacea, peripheral keratitis, Lasik complication, conjunctival surgery, ultraviolet injury

12.1 Introduction

Pterygium is a relatively common occurrence in our aging surgical population. There are a variety of scenarios in which a surgical patient may present with a pterygium, and it is worth looking at these individually and customize a surgical strategy for each targeting an optimal outcome.

An overview of potential patient presentations includes the following:

a) Pterygium as a presenting problem that is primary, isolated, and the sole problem with respect to potential upcoming surgery.
b) Pterygium is the presenting and primary problem, but the patient has other nonsurgical *ocular* concerns that are best addressed in the perioperative period to ensure successful recovery and long-term outcome.
c) Pterygium is the presenting and primary problem, but the patient has other nonsurgical *non-ocular* concerns that are best addressed in the perioperative period to ensure successful recovery and long-term outcome.
d) Pterygium as a presenting surgical problem is primary, but the patient has other ophthalmic surgical concerns that are imminent, concentric, or in need of simultaneous surgery in the same session.

e) Pterygium is present as an incidental finding on a patient presenting for *elective* corneal, cataract, refractive, or glaucoma surgery.
f) Pterygium is present as an incidental finding on a patient presenting for *nonelective* surgery that may involve trauma, endophthalmitis, retinal detachment, chemical injury, or some other emergency.

Let us look at each of these scenarios individually as we prioritize proper management of the pterygium, which is integral to optimizing the ocular surface essential for preserving ocular health, maintaining quality vision, and achieving success in most aspects of modern ophthalmic and particularly anterior segment surgery.

Our "mental checklist" for each of these scenarios prior to any intervention or surgical procedure will ask how this might impact the patient in the following ways:

a) Structural integrity of the eye.
b) Transmission of light/optical pathway.
c) Refracting or focusing of light.
d) Patient comfort.
e) Patient appearance.
f) Patient perception.

Furthermore, it is important to have an understanding of the factors that brought about the development of the pterygium, such as genetic and environmental factors, previous surgery, or trauma. David Paton, MD, is credited with relating that a pterygium on the eye can be thought of similar to the callus on the hand of the farmer. A pterygium is more likely to recur if the ocular surface is re-exposed to the ongoing insult that brought it about in the first place.

12.2 Pterygium: Primary, Isolated, Sole Problem

For the patient presenting with a pterygium as a surgical problem that is primary, isolated, and is the sole problem with respect to potential upcoming surgery, this is relatively straightforward (▶ Fig. 12.1 and ▶ Fig. 12.2). Meticulous resection includes leaving as smooth as possible the corneal

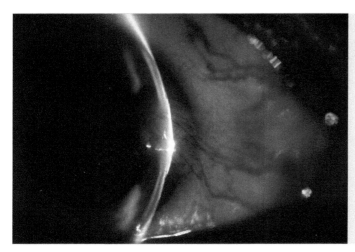

Fig. 12.1 Pterygium encroaching on pupillary margin.

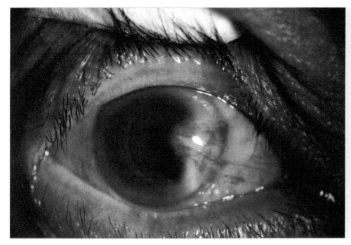

Fig. 12.2 Visually significant chronic pterygium.

surface. The Algerbrush diamond pterygium burr is a technique that the author seldom advocates, as a meticulous dissection is usually superior. The author never uses an antimetabolite on a primary surgical pterygium procedure. Conjunctival flaps, amniotic membrane, and conjunctival grafts all tend to do well in milder cases compliant with respect to reducing and avoiding future ultraviolet (UV) exposure. Conjunctival grafts appear to be superior in the more aggressive and recurrent cases.

12.3 Primary Pterygium Complicated by Additional Ocular Concerns

These patients are very common and require additional attention to ensure proper healing. Local problems may include dry eye or ocular rosacea.

Delayed healing and disease recurrence is more likely to occur in these patients. Addressing dryness, meibomian gland dysfunction (MGD), and exposure prior to surgery will pay dividends when it comes to healing after the surgery and long-term success.

With respect to the ocular form of rosacea, a few additional comments are worth mentioning. Ocular involvement of rosacea is not uncommon but, on occasion, can be easily missed when the ocular involvement is much greater than the cutaneous component. Ocular involvement may appear as bilateral, commonly asymmetric, and on occasion, unilateral. Active keratitis is frequently misdiagnosed as herpes simplex keratitis. Corneal neovascularization can be quite aggressive, and all of this can complicate pterygium before and after surgery. Proactively addressing this not only helps in the perioperative period but also reduces

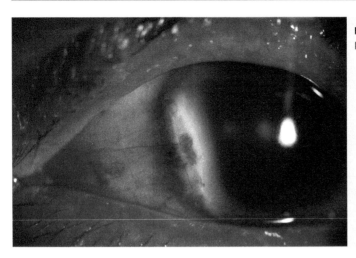

Fig. 12.3 Marginal degeneration with pterygium and pigmentary changes.

complications such as lipid keratopathy in the long run. A nickel allergy is a marker for patients prone to ocular rosacea. Patients, particularly female patients, may have a history of problems wearing jewelry made with 10 ct gold. For example, 10 ct earrings are made with a nickel alloy that many rosacea patients are unfortunately allergic to; it turns their ear lobes green.

Early ocular cicatricial pemphigoid (OCP) and other forms of cicatrizing conjunctivitis may be aggravated by pterygium surgery and may impact the decision to undergo surgery. Surgery in these patients may require a prolonged course of corticosteroids postoperatively.

Glaucoma patients bring special consideration as topical glaucoma medications are somewhat toxic and irritating to the ocular surface, which may impact healing and pterygium recurrence. Additionally, previous or future glaucoma surgery may be impacted by the extent of conjunctival resection that accompanies pterygium surgery. Furthermore, these patients need IOP monitoring more closely, taking into consideration the postoperative use of topical corticosteroids after pterygium surgery.

12.4 Primary Pterygium Complicated by Additional Nonocular Concerns

Another concern that can contribute to complex pterygium management is the patient who presents with a history of peripheral noninfectious keratitis—found in patients who develop ocular involvement of an underlying autoimmune disease. There are many conditions (rheumatoid arthritis, scleroderma, polyarteritis nodosa, Wegener's granulomatosis, and Mooren's ulceration) where inflammation and tissue loss may result in a pterygium in the healing response (▶ Fig. 12.3). There may be minimal tissue support underneath the pterygium, and these patients should be approached cautiously realizing the autoimmune process could recur. Furthermore, in some of these more severe cases, the pterygium may be part of a healing process that is lending tissue support. Avoiding surgery may be the best approach in these complex patients as a surgical approach will likely require a corneal patch graft. In these cases, the eye is diseased, and pterygium growth is a response to inflammation and healing. It is important to make sure that the patient has been fully evaluated and is under optimal systemic management before tackling the ocular surface surgically. A very important consideration here is the patient who has recurrent pterygium who may also have undergone a procedure that used an antimetabolite or even radiation in the distant past that can further complicate these eyes with perforation or poor healing.

12.5 Combined Pterygium Surgery

A common scenario would be a patient presenting for pterygium surgery, but it is also apparent that they concomitantly have epithelial basement membrane dystrophy (EBMD) or Salzmann's nodular dystrophy involving the cornea in addition to pterygium. Some of these patients will have a

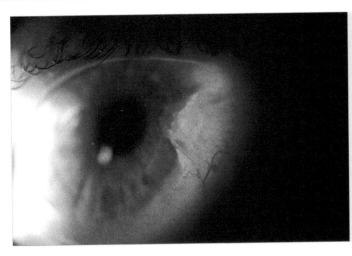

Fig. 12.4 Pterygium with Salzmann's nodular degeneration at the leading edge.

Salzmann's nodule at the leading head of the pterygium (photo). Patients having pterygium with these types of corneal involvement are best managed with combining pterygium surgery with superficial keratectomy and, when appropriate, phototherapeutic keratectomy (PTK) for a more complete treatment to "polish" the ocular surface for healing that leads to an optimized ocular surface and outcome. Anticipated glaucoma surgery should take into account the preservation of conjunctiva. Anticipated cataract surgery should take into account the goal of a smooth, stable ocular surface allowing reliable intraocular lens calculations.

When pterygium coexists with forms of ocular disease, such as EBMD or Salzmann's nodular degeneration (▶ Fig. 12.4), the clinical and surgical strategy is often more involved and patients are often pre-treated with oral doxycycline particularly if they have MGD (▶ Fig. 12.5). Punctal plugs, serum tears, oral vitamin C, amniotic membrane, and temporary tarsorrhaphy are all considerations for these special cases where stem cell reserve is guarded. Dry eye disease is increasing in our aging patients. This is an important consideration in our presurgical patients, particularly in the pre-cataract patient, where successful management of complex ocular surface cases will permit more surgical options with greater likelihood of success when cataract surgery is eventually performed.

12.6 Anterior Segment Surgery with Incidental Pterygium

When a patient presents for elective eye surgery but also has a pterygium that is not the primary problem, surgical options include the following:

a) Address the primary problem and avoid disturbing the pterygium.
b) Address both the primary problem and the pterygium in a single surgical procedure.
c) Address the primary problem and, if necessary, the pterygium in a staged procedure.

The first option might be seen in a variety of scenarios that would include the individual who simply is not bothered by the pterygium, and the pterygium is not going to adversely impact the outcome of the primary procedure.

Poorly controlled glaucoma requiring filtering or a shunt procedure would take priority over an early pterygium, and additional conjunctival surgery would not be ideal in this scenario. OCP is another condition that can be "stirred up" with the type of surgery that would involve pterygium resection. Managing the primary problem along with the pterygium in a single surgical procedure ([b], above) is very reasonable in non-refractive procedures presenting in combination with a pterygium. A mild pterygium that is periodically red, inflamed, causing discomfort, but not impacting the quality of measuring the ocular surface could also be resected in combination with cataract surgery or corneal transplantation. A more significant pterygium removed in a staged procedure ([c], above) and allowed to heal would allow for better measurements for intraocular lens (IOL) calculations prior to cataract surgery. This would be the case for a variety of procedures seeking an optimal refractive outcome.

We have examination and imaging techniques that allow us to more precisely determine how much a pterygium is contributing to astigmatism.

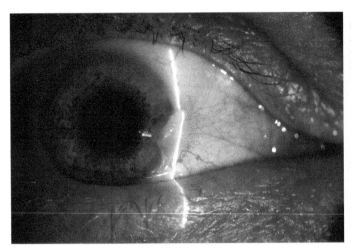

Fig. 12.5 Nasal pterygium with associated spheroidal degeneration sometimes called an amyloid pterygium.

In the cataract patient, it is important to recognize that a toric IOL could become a liability if the pterygium progresses or is removed in the future. In these cases, the pterygium should be removed first with a technique that reduces future recurrence. Once the ocular surface is stable, it is then reasonable to remeasure the IOL calculations and look for the best options for each patient individually. Furthermore, I discourage treating astigmatism caused by a pterygium with an astigmatic keratotomy (limbal relaxing incision [LRI]). This would be like finding a car tire with an air leak and treating it by letting air out of the other three tires. Whenever possible, treat the problem where the problem is located.

An example of a staged procedure that would postpone pterygium removal would be a patient with a traumatic corneal laceration where the emphasis is placed on the more emergent procedure and deprioritizing the pterygium as an elective procedure.

Full thickness penetrating keratoplasty (PK) is a special case as this may fail through immunologic rejection, and long-term failure from ocular surface disease is even more prevalent. These are cases where concomitant pterygium has a role in managing and optimizing the ocular surface. A partial thickness endothelial keratoplasty procedure (Descemet's stripping automated endothelial keratoplasty [DSAEK], Descemet's membrane endothelial keratoplasty [DMEK], and pre-Descemet's endothelial keratoplasty [PDEK]) is greatly preferred in cases primarily involving endothelial dysfunction, and the presence of a pterygium makes these newer procedures even more appealing. Further surgical consideration is necessary while performing corneal transplantation using a vacuum trephine to prepare the recipient corneal bed. In these cases, the obturating ring of the vacuum trephine may not be able to achieve and sustain adequate suction.

Another surgical consideration in patients having a pterygium is that femtosecond lasers used to create Lasik flaps and also used in cataract surgery may not be able to engage adequate suction to stabilize the eye and enable a safe progression of surgery.

Deep anterior lamellar keratoplasty (DALK) is increasingly popular as a procedure to manage anterior corneal scarring. While a minor pterygium could probably be managed during the primary procedure, a more severe pterygium would be better managed in a staged procedure allowing healing before performing a DALK procedure.

12.7 Complex Eye Surgery with Incidental Pterygium

Another situation might include a serious emergency, and the additional procedure involving the pterygium is just not an immediate concern unless a laceration is extending through an existing pterygium. An acute retinal detachment or intraocular foreign body that can be addressed without adding any additional complexity is offered by pterygium surgery.

12.8 Additional Considerations in the Surgical Management of Pterygium

The importance of the ocular surface for proper transmission and refraction of light entering the eye has elevated importance in patients desiring newer technologies, such as multifocal intraocular lenses. In addition, it is not uncommon for patients with visual complaints that seem out of proportion to their Snellen acuity. While patients may see 20/20 or better under artificial "Snellen" conditions—in a dark, quiet room, looking at maximum contrast black letters on a white background—this may not properly reflect how they are functioning in the real world experiencing a loss of contrast and glare intolerance. The ocular surface may be underappreciated in this regard when the patient has a reasonable Snellen acuity or if the focus is on some other aspect of the eye. The ocular surface is increasingly recognized as an essential component in quality patient care.

While numerous new methods for evaluating and documenting the severity of a pterygium are available, one of the most overlooked methods is the very simple method of utilizing qualitative wavefront analysis—using retinoscopy. This technique is frequently more revealing than many of our more sophisticated methods, and is particularly helpful in decision making while thinking about the timing of cataract surgery in the presence of a pterygium. Retinoscopy is readily available and is especially helpful in patients offering visual complaints that appear out of proportion to the findings on examination.

While a genetic predisposition to pterygium has been reported,[1,2] a special subgroup of pterygium is associated with another condition thought to be inherited—EBMD, anterior membrane dystrophy, Cogan's microcystic dystrophy, map-dot-finger-print dystrophy—where the underlying genetic problem is at the level of the hemidesmosome resulting in several phenotypes, including EBMD. These patients may also exhibit recurrent corneal erosion syndrome, contact lens intolerance, loose epithelium during eye surgery including Lasik (particularly with a mechanical microkeratome), Salzmann's nodular degeneration, and a combined Salzmann's nodule with a pterygium (Fig. 12.4, Fig. 12.5). EBMD may be very subtle, requiring much more than casual examination of the cornea using slit-lamp biomicroscopy. Direct focal illumination, indirect retroillumination, and scleral scatter are the three best illumination techniques for detecting subtle EBMD. Fluorescein stain may also be used to help detect what some people refer to as "negative staining" when an elevated area breaks through the pooled layer of stain.

Whether pterygium is the primary or associated concern, it is important to consider this while developing a surgical strategy that targets optimal patient care.

References

[1] Kau HC, Tsai CC, Hsu WM, Liu JH, Wei YH. Genetic polymorphism of hOGG1 and risk of pterygium in Chinese. Eye (Lond). 2004; 18(6):635–639

[2] Anguria P, Kitinya J, Ntuli S, Carmichael T. The role of heredity in pterygium development. Int J Ophthalmol. 2014; 7(3): 563–573

13 Complications of Pterygium Surgery

Dhivya Ashok Kumar, Soosan Jacob, Ashvin Agarwal, and Amar Agarwal

Abstract

Pterygium is a degenerative condition with fibro-vascular growth on the conjunctiva that has been noted to be common in hot and dry climate countries. Surgical excision is often performed in symptomatic cases, which include the complete excision with conjunctival autograft with fibrin glue or sutures. The common complications of surgery include hemorrhage, recurrence, graft-related complications, scleral thinning, and scar. Application of amniotic membrane graft and use of antifibrotic agents can also reduce recurrence.

Keywords: pterygium excision, surgical complications, hemorrhage, recurrence

13.1 Introduction

The surgical methods of pterygium removal vary from the simplest bare sclera excision to sophisticated keratoplastics and transplantation procedures. The treatment of pterygium does not conclude with mechanical removal alone. The postoperative complications are not uncommon in pterygium excision. These can be due to the initial surgical technique, adjuvant drugs used such as antimetabolites, sutures-related, or the postoperative medications. Recurrence and residual scarring is commonly experienced in clinical practice. This can be seen in early or late postoperative period. Vision-threatening complications, such as corneal perforation, melting, and postoperative infections, though rare, are also reported. Hence, in this section, we have mainly focused on the postoperative complications and their management.

13.2 Complications after Pterygium Excision

The complications in pterygium surgery can be classified as intraoperative, early postoperative, and late postoperative.

13.2.1 Intraoperative Complications

Hemorrhage

Excessive bleeding can occur in highly vascularized thick pterygium. Identifying the bleeder and doing meticulous cautery on the blood vessel can reduce the incidence. Avoid holding the fleshy part of the pterygium with traumatic toothed forceps directly on the blood vessel. Hemorrhage can also happen in inflamed pterygium; therefore, inflamed pterygium has to be controlled by anti-inflammatory agents or low potent steroid before surgery. Hemorrhage can occur from the scleral bed after excision of the pterygium, and this has to be controlled by good cautious diathermy.

Scleral Lamella Removal

While excising the pterygium, the surgeon can inadvertently excise the underlying scleral lamella also. If the excised layer is thin, it will not cause significant problems postoperatively. However, if the depth of lamella is more, there can be scleral thinning and uveal exposure later. Hence, we recommend intraoperative visualization of the base and the posterior surface of the pterygium during excision.

Excess Cautery of Sclera

In case of excessive bleeding which obscures the visibility, the surgeon may cauterize the sclera along with the blood vessel. This may lead to scleral thinning and perforation. Hence, it is always required to visualize the zone of cautery and to utilize minimal power.

Corneal Damage

While doing the lamellar dissection of the pterygium on the corneal surface, the crescent blade can go deeper and cause disruption of normal corneal uninvolved stroma. This can rarely cause perforation and corneal scarring postoperatively. Hence, surgeons should take precaution not to dissect deeper, and a preoperative anterior segment optical coherence tomography can aid in such situation to determine the depth of dissection.

13.2.2 Immediate Postoperative Complications

Reactionary Hemorrhage

Reactionary hemorrhage occurs in the postoperative period due to dislodge of clot in the blood vessel, which induces it to rebleed spontaneously (▶ Fig. 13.1). Pressure bandage usually controls it. Patients with systemic hypertension should continue their antihypertensive medications to prevent rebleed.

Conjunctival Chemosis

Conjunctival chemosis can be seen in few patients which resolves spontaneously.

Conjunctival Graft Edema

Graft edema may be seen in the early postoperative period; however, it resolves with topical treatment.

Conjunctival Recession

The conjunctiva may recede in the early postoperative period and expose the underlying sclera (▶ Fig. 13.2). This can occur due to tight conjunctival suturing or inadequate conjunctival closure. If the exposed region is more and there is scleral thinning, it will require repeat conjunctival closure by autograft or amniotic membrane graft.

Graft Reversal

Conjunctival autograft or amniotic membrane graft can turn or give way from the scleral bed with one end of the graft hanging (▶ Fig. 13.3). This can happen when the conjunctiva has not been properly

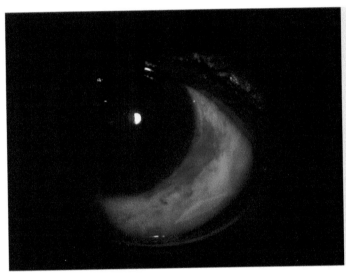

Fig. 13.1 Hemorrhage below the amniotic membrane graft in the immediate postoperative period.

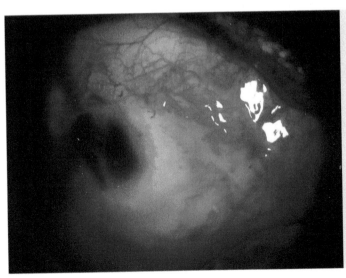

Fig. 13.2 Conjunctiva receded in the immediate postoperative period.

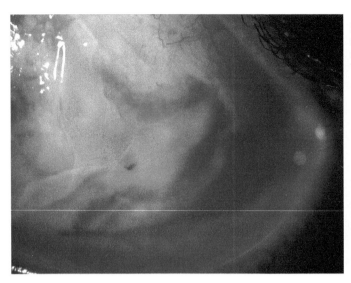

Fig. 13.3 Amniotic membrane graft slipped from the underlying sclera surface in the immediate postoperative period.

adhered with fibrin glue, or if the sutures are loose. The possible reasons for the poor adhesion are due to improper application of tissue glue or sutures. The patient should be taken again to OR, for repositioning of the graft to be performed.

Hematoma

Hematoma below the graft may occur due to persistent bleeding because of improper hemostasis. In this case, the graft is examined under microscope, and hematoma is evacuated under block.

Localized Epithelial Defect

The localized epithelial defect is seen in almost all patients on day 1 of postoperative period, which heals within 24 hours.

Corneal Scar

Corneal scar, either a macular or nebular opacity, depending upon the depth of corneal involvement may be observed from the immediate postoperative period. Excess scar or deep opacity may require lamellar keratoplasty later.

13.3 Late Complications

13.3.1 Recurrence

One of the major limitations of pterygium excision is the high rate of postoperative recurrence. The recurrence time ranges from months to years.

Increased fibroblastic activity is a well-established finding in recurrent pterygia. Recurrent pterygium is more difficult to treat than primary pterygium because it is often accompanied by increased conjunctival inflammation and accelerated corneal involvement. Partial limbal stem cell deficiency and coexisting inflammation might be one of the etiologies for recurrent pterygia. The recurrence rate was 10.9% (primary), 37.5% (recurrence), and 14.8% (all pterygium) after pterygium excision with amniotic membrane graft in a study by Prabhasawat et al.[1] Conjunctival autograft showed a recurrence of 2.6% (primary), 9.1% (recurrence), and 4.9% (all pterygium).

13.3.2 Treatment

Intraoperative use of antimetabolites, namely mitomycin C (MMC), reduces the risk of recurrence.[2,3,4] Lee et al has reported that MMC effects are stronger in recurrent pterygium than those with primary cells.[5] Conjunctival autograft with pterygium excision is known to show less recurrence and is the first choice of surgical treatment.[1,6] Amniotic membrane is a good alternate choice to reduce recurrence in advanced cases with bilateral heads or in patients who might need glaucoma surgery later.[6] The postoperative instillation of MMC 0.02% (0.2 mg/mL) eye drops twice daily for 5 days following excision of primary pterygium has been used to reduce recurrence.[7] Topical bevacizumab (5 mg/mL) twice a day has shown to delay the recurrence in impending recurrent pterygia.[8] Single-dose beta-irradiation after bare sclera surgery in the postoperative period is a simple, effective, and safe treatment that reduces the risk of primary pterygium recurrence. An Sr-90 eye applicator is used to deliver 2500 cGy to the sclera surface at a dose rate of between 200 and 250 cGy/min.[9]

13.3.3 Complications Due to Use of Mitomycin C

Topical

MMC is an antimetabolite agent produced by a strain of *Streptomyces caespitosus.* It inhibits synthesis of deoxyribonucleic acid (DNA), ribonucleic acid (RNA), and proteins. This drug is referred to as "radio-mimetic" as its action mimics that of ionizing radiation. Topical 0.02% eye drops have been known to cause ocular complications, such as superficial punctate keratitis, avascularized sclera, and pyogenic granuloma. Ocular discomfort and lacrimation are some of the common complaints. MMC 0.5 mg/mL has also been used after pterygium excision and beta-irradiation, which leads to complications such as scleromalacia, scleral ulcer, and cataract.[10]

Intraoperative Mitomycin C

Scleral dellen is an early postoperative complication of bare sclera technique with MMC owing to delayed conjunctival wound closure.[11] Treated sclera may become white or "porcelainized" due to destroyed vessels and remain so forever. It has been reported that it is due to the drug's effect on multipotential cells and the rapidly proliferating cells of vascular endothelium.[12] Complications including temporary and prolonged discomfort, tearing, hyperemia, subconjunctival hemorrhage, wound dehiscence, and pigment accumulation were also noted with a single dose of intraoperative MMC by Anduze and Burnett.[13] Hence, it is recommended that only high-risk pterygia should receive MMC. Conjunctiva should cover the sclera up to the limbus and thereby preventing migration of MMC. They concluded that a single dose of 0.5 mg/mL subconjunctivally gives the same results as multiple drops do, but with far less morbidity.

13.3.4 Suture-Related Inflammation

Suture-related inflammation is commonly seen with polyglactin sutures. Proper postoperative antibiotic applications can reduce it. Some surgeons prefer to use monofilament nylon for suturing the autograft due to an increase in inflammation with Vicryl sutures.

13.3.5 Tenon's Cyst

This can occur in eyes in which the Tenon's layer was exposed. Excision of the cyst with complete closure is recommended. Improper conjunctival autograft separation, in which the conjunctiva is harvested with thick Tenon's layer, may be a risk factor for such complication.

13.3.6 Diplopia and Squint

Scarring and excessive fibrosis in region of pterygium or in the conjunctiva can lead to restriction of extraocular movements and diplopia. The patients with tendencies for keloid formation and hypertrophic scar are at high risk of developing such complication. Excess scarring can occasionally cause restrictive strabismus. In such cases, scar exploration and release of fibrosis are usually performed.

13.3.7 Scleral Complications

Scleral ulceration was present in 51 eyes on a long-term follow-up by Tarr and Constable.[14] Scleral thinning with perforation can also happen as a late complication. Excessive cautery to the scleral bed should be avoided as it can induce scleral thinning (▶ Fig. 13.4). Overenthusiastic use of antimetabolites can lead to scleral complications. Pseudomonas endophthalmitis occurred in four patients with scleral ulceration.[15] He observed that beta irradiation to prevent recurrence of pterygia is a significant cause of iatrogenic ocular disease. Patients with scleral thinning can be put on copious lubricants to improve ocular surface healing. Nonhealing scleral thinning and impending scleral perforation will require patch graft or amniotic membrane graft.

13.3.8 Corneal Perforation

Pterygium excision can lead to corneal thinning. We have seen corneal perforation in two eyes with a history of excessive straining after pterygium excision. One patient had intraoperative MMC, and the other patient had excessive scarring. Patch graft was performed for both patients. Corneoscleral perforation with iris prolapse was reported by Dadeya and Fatima[16] after intraoperative MMC.

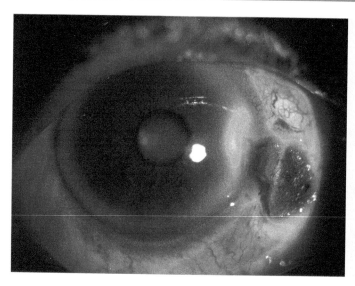

Fig. 13.4 Scleral thinning after pterygium surgery.

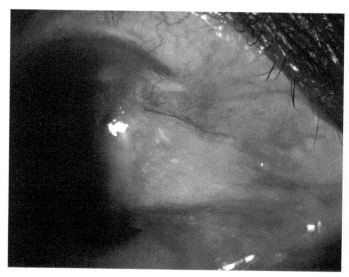

Fig. 13.5 Thick fleshy pterygium involving cornea has potential for scar formation.

13.3.9 Residual Corneal Scar

Deep pterygium involving the cornea can leave scar after excision (▶ Fig. 13.5). Improper lamellar dissection and patients with keloid tendencies can have significant scar formation. Eyes with deep corneal involvement can be combined with lamellar keratoplasty during the primary procedure itself.

13.3.10 Lens Changes

Radiation-induced cataract occurred in three eyes in a study by Tarr and Constable.[14] Sectorial lens opacities with normal visual acuity was seen in 19 eyes in their follow-up.

13.3.11 Miscellaneous

Ptosis, symblepharon, and iris atrophy were also seen after pterygium excision with irradiation.

13.4 Conclusion

Complications are inevitable in any surgical procedure; however, prevention and managing make the difference in the functional outcome. Meticulous following of surgical steps, avoiding excess cautery, and good postoperative follow-up should invariably improve the success rate after pterygium surgery. Use of newer adjunctive methods, such as amniotic membrane or conjunctival autograft, and cautious topical use of MMC can aid in minimizing the recurrences.

References

[1] Prabhasawat P, Barton K, Burkett G, Tseng SC. Comparison of conjunctival autografts, amniotic membrane grafts, and primary closure for pterygium excision. Ophthalmology. 1997; 104(6):974–985

[2] Donnenfeld ED, Perry HD, Fromer S, Doshi S, Solomon R, Biser S. Subconjunctival mitomycin C as adjunctive therapy before pterygium excision. Ophthalmology. 2003; 110(5):1012–1016

[3] Frucht-Pery J, Siganos CS, Ilsar M. Intraoperative application of topical mitomycin C for pterygium surgery. Ophthalmology. 1996; 103(4):674–677

[4] Frucht-Pery J, Ilsar M. The use of low-dose mitomycin C for prevention of recurrent pterygium. Ophthalmology. 1994; 101(4):759–762

[5] Lee JS, Oum BS, Lee SH. Mitomycin c influence on inhibition of cellular proliferation and subsequent synthesis of type I collagen and laminin in primary and recurrent pterygia. Ophthalmic Res. 2001; 33(3):140–146

[6] Luanratanakorn P, Ratanapakorn T, Suwan-Apichon O, Chuck RS. Randomised controlled study of conjunctival autograft versus amniotic membrane graft in pterygium excision. Br J Ophthalmol. 2006; 90(12):1476–1480

[7] Rachmiel R, Leiba H, Levartovsky S. Results of treatment with topical mitomycin C 0.02% following excision of primary pterygium. Br J Ophthalmol. 1995; 79(3):233–236

[8] Fallah MR, Khosravi K, Hashemian MN, Beheshtnezhad AH, Rajabi MT, Gohari M. Efficacy of topical bevacizumab for inhibiting growth of impending recurrent pterygium. Curr Eye Res. 2010; 35(1):17–22

[9] Jürgenliemk-Schulz IM, Hartman LJ, Roesink JM, et al. Prevention of pterygium recurrence by postoperative single-dose beta-irradiation: a prospective randomized clinical double-blind trial. Int J Radiat Oncol Biol Phys. 2004; 59(4):1138–1147

[10] Saifuddin S, el Zawawi A. Scleral changes due to mitomycin C after pterygium excision: a report of two cases. Indian J Ophthalmol. 1995; 43(2):75–76

[11] Tsai YY, Lin JM, Shy JD. Acute scleral thinning after pterygium excision with intraoperative mitomycin C: a case report of scleral dellen after bare sclera technique and review of the literature. Cornea. 2002; 21(2):227–229

[12] Rubinfeld RS, Pfister RR, Stein RM, et al. Serious complications of topical mitomycin-C after pterygium surgery. Ophthalmology. 1992; 99(11):1647–1654

[13] Anduze AL, Burnett JM. Indications for and complications of mitomycin-C in pterygium surgery. Ophthalmic Surg Lasers. 1996; 27(8):667–673

[14] Tarr KH, Constable IJ. Late complications of pterygium treatment. Br J Ophthalmol. 1980; 64(7):496–505

[15] Jain V, Shome D, Natarajan S, Narverkar R. Surgically induced necrotizing scleritis after pterygium surgery with conjunctival autograft. Cornea. 2008; 27(6):720–721

[16] Dadeya S, Fatima S. Comeoscleral perforation after pterygium excision and intraoperative mitomycin C. Ophthalmic Surg Lasers Imaging. 2003; 34(2):146–148

14 Complex Pterygium Surgery and Complication Management to Cosmetic Endpoints

Arun C. Gulani and Aaishwariya A. Gulani

Abstract

Pterygium complications and complex ptergyium surgery can also be designed using minimalistic and even staged, least interventional approaches to deliver a cosmetic and visually enhanced outcome using complexity and recAmniotic grafts can be used in a full-spectrum oc-ular surface and corneal disorders for aesthetically and visually excellent outcomes. Such disorders in-clude corneal surface instability, recurrent corneal erosions, Lasik complications, Salzmann s nodules, and anterior corneal dystrophies.

Keywords: Reccurent Pterygium, Pterygium complications, scleral melts, Pterygium surgery, ProKera, corneal scars, SPARKLE, lamellar keratoplasty, scleral patch, stem cells, SLET, amniotic graft, Gulani

14.1 Introduction

Following my previous chapter regarding a relentless mindset to deliver pterygium patients an eye that is cosmetically enhanced (▶ Fig. 14.1) and visually improved,[1,2,3] I shall in this chapter discuss my experience with complex pterygium cases and complications.

Once again, I want to reiterate the "mindset."

Aggressive pterygia, recurrent pterygia, symblepharon, corneal scars, scleral melts, etc. should be approached with the unshakable desire to not only restore the ocular anatomy and fix the complication but to also deliver an eye to emmetropic vision and a cosmetic outcome.

With a worldwide referral base for complex pterygia and pinguecula complication cases, I have condensed my observations and approach over nearly three decades to share in this chapter.

Personally, I have seen < 0.5% recurrence rate over 16 years with my sutureless amniotic technique despite doing very complex pterygia. Nevertheless, I have witnessed and experienced some adverse outcomes as stated before including self-limiting ones, such as pyogenic granulomas, mild scleral thinning, and subamniotic hemorrhage (▶ Fig. 14.2) while also having been responsible for

a case each of muscle adhesion, accidental graft displacement, and pupil deformation.

This only underscores the fact that I insist every patient verbalize full understanding of this surgery despite the wonderful results they may have read about or reviewed in their research as well as make every surgeon accountable for their responsibility toward outcomes which in many cases could be patient or incident dependent.

Once again, I must first emphasize that the mindset associated with treating recurrent ptergia and associated complications is the same as when dealing with the virgin pterygium surgery.

Surgeons should not adopt the notion that the previous surgeon did a bad job, or that they are now trying to help a patient and therefore aim for a mediocre outcome. Rather, the mindset should be the same as when treating the primary pterygium with the expectation of achieving outstanding cosmetic outcomes on the next postoperative day that will remain stable in the future. Every step should not only correct the problem but also enhance the appearance of the eye and possibly improve vision too.

When correcting recurrences and complications arising in pterygia/pinguecula surgery, I have suggested four facets that surgeons must consider[4,5,6]:

1. The recurrence and/or complications of the lesion itself.
2. Associated conditions, such as fornix shortening, corneal and conjunctival scarring, symblepharon, ischemia, or scleral melts.
3. Predisposing factor for such a recurrence/complication.
4. Plan an endpoint that will allow that patient to avail of options for vision corrective surgery, that is, Lasik, premium cataract surgery, etc.

Regardless of the expertise of the surgeon who performed the initial surgery, complications can develop that require devising a treatment plan with realistic expectations for the patient, but without lowering our own desire to achieve excellence.

I always presume and reiterate to patients that their initial surgeon did the best they could of removing the lesion; the goals of the second

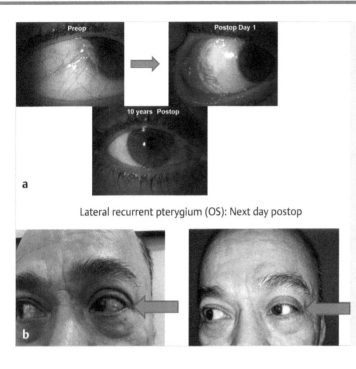

Lateral recurrent pterygium (OS): Next day postop

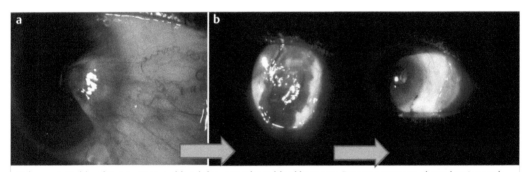

Sub-amniotic blood in a patient on blood thinners who rubbed her eyes. Day one post-op, cleared at 1 month.

Fig. 14.2 (a,b) Self-limiting subamniotic hemorrhage.

surgeon now are to pick up the baton and take it to the end zone by beautifying the eye, correcting the comorbidity of associated problems, and enhancing vision.

14.2 Resecting Recurrent Lesions

In summary of my previous book chapter where I have described my "iceberg" surgical concept in detail using sutureless, amniotic graft along with mitomycin C (MMC) application and glue, we should keep the mentality of minimalistic dissection and have a single goal of finding the bare sclera by careful and gentle cut down through the recurrent scar tissue.[7,8]

The first surgeon has usually done a nice job of preparing a clear/bare sclera waiting to be discovered. Once we reach that plane, you can take a breath as the most difficult part is over. In most cases, now the rest of the scariform tissue lifts off like a "plate of armor" from the underlying sclera.

Following this approach, there is minimal bleeding (bleeding usually occurs when surgeons chase the scar tissue from different approaches and cut into it causing multiple planes with a messy and distorted anatomy that further complicates surgical steps).

In majority of recurrent cases that are referred to me, I will find the original pterygium only partially removed; therefore, I insist on complete removal of primary pterygium as a basis of consistent success in virgin eyes. Follow the surgical technique as outlined to completion including MMC application and Tisseel glue along with amniotic graft reconstruction (▶ Fig. 14.3 and ▶ Fig. 14.4).

14.3 Focusing on Associated Pathology

After the mass of the pterygium is removed, the surgeon should consider the anatomy and methods to improve the ocular appearance and address the associated comorbidities.

One such adjustment is forming the fornices. This is done by redeepening and relieving the conjunctival scarring and symblepharon, clearing the corneal area using a number 64 blade without cutting in a smooth rapid fashion, and then applying an amniotic graft to reconstruct the fornix by deepening it and arranging the conjunctiva in an elaborate fashion such that it is cosmetically hidden under the lids, but is functionally viable.

This amniotic membrane can also be used in layers to reinforce the sclera while creating normal

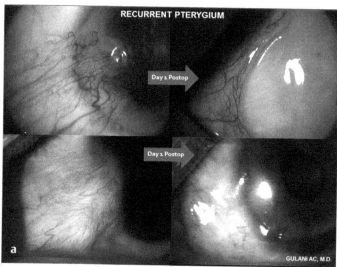

Fig. 14.3 (a,b) Recurrent pterygium excision, next day and long-term the appearance.

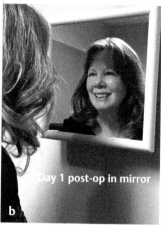

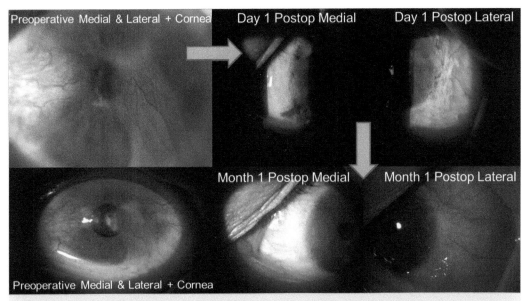

Fig. 14.4 Aggressive bitemporal recurrent pterygium with medial and lateral sutureless AMT and sliding Tenon technique laterally. AMT, amniotic membrane transplantation.

anatomical relations of the ocular surface. The membrane is attached using Tisseel glue (Baxter International). The area of the corneal scar is smoothed, and application of the amniotic membrane can be extended beyond the limbus onto the cornea for better healing. In many of these cases, I use ProKera (Bio-Tissue) or AmbioDisk (Katena) on the day after the surgery.

Sclera melts are another possible complication of pterygium surgery; some of these are self resolving while others require a tissue intervention, such as lamellar cornea, conjunctival, or Tenon's pedicles, and amniotic graft reconstruction. In severe cases, I also use Tutoplast with amniotic graft combination to further reconstruct and strengthen the sclera (▶ Fig. 14.5, ▶ Fig. 14.6, ▶ Fig. 14.7, ▶ Fig. 14.8, ▶ Fig. 14.9, ▶ Fig. 14.10c).

The Tenon's pedicle can be used to supply vascularity to a usually ischemic sclera, and the lamellar cornea can be used in superficial scleral thinnings and glued in place, so we have a cosmetically appealing endpoint.

Granulomas can occur in some cases too and can resolve by themselves, with steroid eye drops or gentle cautery excision.

In extensive and deeper involvements of sclera, I have used Tutoplast and tried to always keep it least bulky (keeping in mind that though these are salvage cases, still can we keep the extraocular movement and appearance the best we can). Do not hesitate to take anchor sutures if needed by involving surrounding anatomical leverages to strengthen the structures affected. These cases can look cosmetically appealing the next day after surgery and remain that way for years to come. Clearing and strengthening are the main objectives though cosmesis and vision are our relentless desire. Complications of the I-Brite procedures popularized on the West Coast when referred to me have also been successfully addressed using these principles (▶ Fig. 14.11a–d).

Corneal scars can be easily addressed using ProKera technology with lamellar keratectomy and MMC application (▶ Fig. 14.12 and ▶ Fig. 14.13).

In cases with residual corneal scars, we can apply Corneoplastique principles to use the excimer laser in a refractive mode and bring these patients to emmetropic vision, a dream outcome for such cases, which had relegated their future to a cosmetically poor appearing eye with glasses or

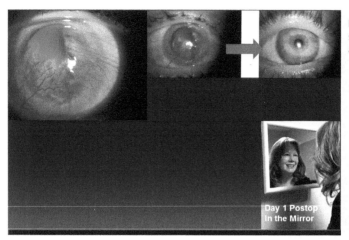

Fig. 14.5 Recurrent, lateral pterygium sclera reinforced with Tenon's pedicle anchor.

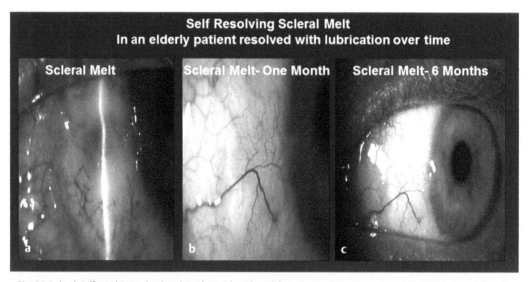

Fig. 14.6 (a-c) Self-resolving scleral melt with good ocular surface management.

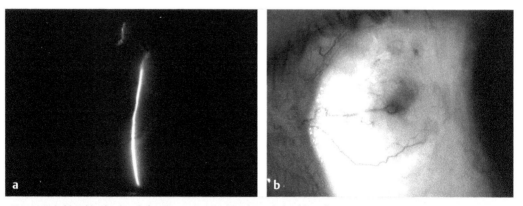

Fig. 14.7 (a,b) Mild scleral melt for observation and backup of glued lamellar cornea.

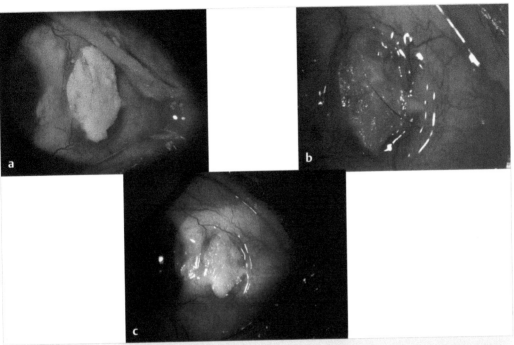

Fig. 14.8 (a-c) Scleral melt with calcification and cheesy deposit with multiple eyelash entrapment referred for surgery. I am observing for now, as the patient is stable with calcific plaque sealing scleral melt and vision 20/20 with good comfort. Do not jump into surgery!

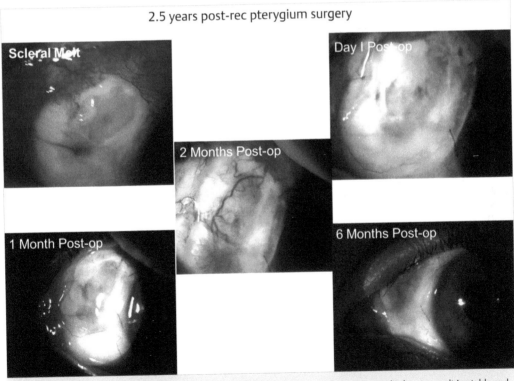

Fig. 14.9 Glued lamellar cornea used to seal scleral melt along with two anchor sutures at limbus to result in stable and cosmetic outcome along with maintaining 20/20 vision. (*continued*)

2.5 years post-rec pterygium surgery

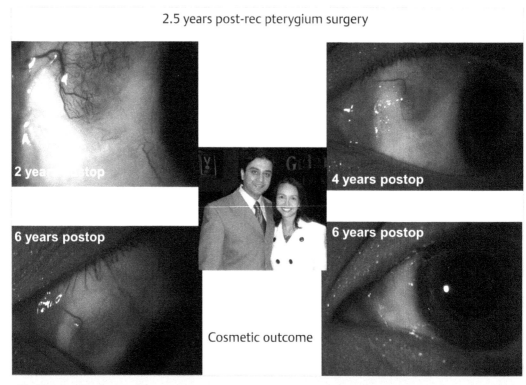

Fig. 14.9 (continued)

contact lenses and limited lifestyle options therein (▶ Fig. 14.14).

14.4 Predisposing Comorbidities

If predisposing conditions, such as rheumatoid arthritis, Sjogren's syndrome, dry eyes, or collagen vascular diseases are present, we must involve the patient's physician for a work-up and management systemically.

In addition, every attempt at surgery raises the chance of recurrence, so we must strive to do it right the first time following principles of the iceberg concept.

This minimalistic, but intensely directed approach results in consistently good results for these patients with its elegant arrangement of tissue. The cosmetic outcomes, high functionality, and improved vision are the final goals of this surgery regardless of the appearance before the surgery. Therefore, recurrent pterygia can be addressed in the same fashion, but with a slightly different approach and the same mindset as the initial surgeries (▶ Fig. 14.15).

Importantly, numerous patients referred to us, in whom I have corrected their complex pterygium and complications, have also undergone subsequent laser vision surgery and premium cataract surgery with excellent visual outcomes, a caveat in today's times. Given the unique nature of my practice that sees a number of patients flying for cosmetic outcomes, their expectations need to be addressed because doing a mediocre job on a case where the pterygium/pinguecula was primary and small, but resulting in a postoperative scar is less tolerable and more agonizing than a recurrence in a complex pterygium case.

This is very much similar to present day premium Lasik or cataract surgery where patients with 20/60 vision and easy cataract expect perfection as opposed to someone with 20/400 vision even if the patient with 20/400 vision may have a more complicated cataract.

This is a price we must pay for our desire to excel for our patients by undertaking this level of commitment, as long as the patients are educated about the fact that complications can occur.

Mastering the art of pterygium and pinguecula surgery to treat emerging cases as well as

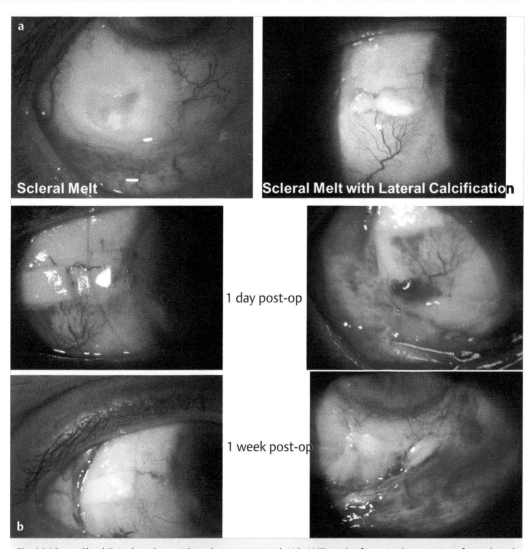

Fig. 14.10 a-c Glued Tutoplast along with anchor sutures used with AMT overlay for smooth separation of muscle and eye movement along with restored integrity, cosmesis, comfort, and future vision correction. AMT, amniotic membrane transplantation. (*continued*)

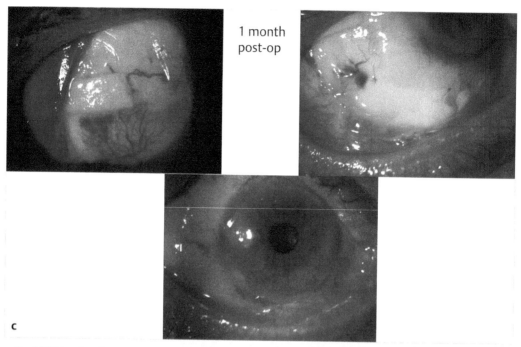

1 month
post-op

c

Fig. 14.10 (*continued*)

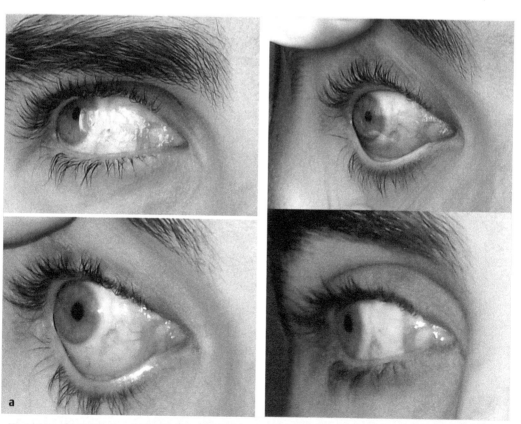

a

Fig. 14.11 a-d Patients referred after I-Brite complications such as these with scleral melts and symptomatic eyes can be rejuvenated by restoring ocular surface stability and comfort using amniotic graft reconstruction to cosmetic outcomes. AMT, amniotic membrane transplantation. (*continued*)

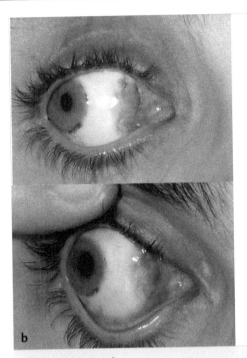
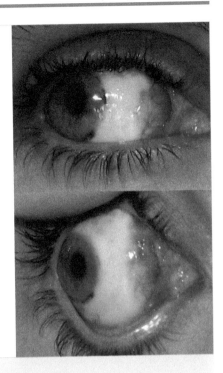

1 week
post-op

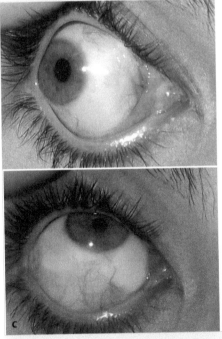

b

Fig. 14.11 (continued)

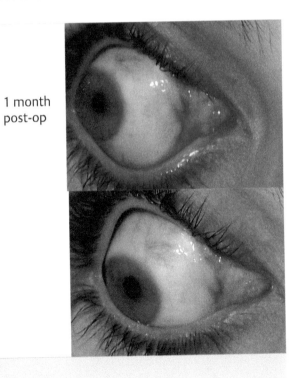

1 month
post-op

c

Fig. 14.11 (continued)

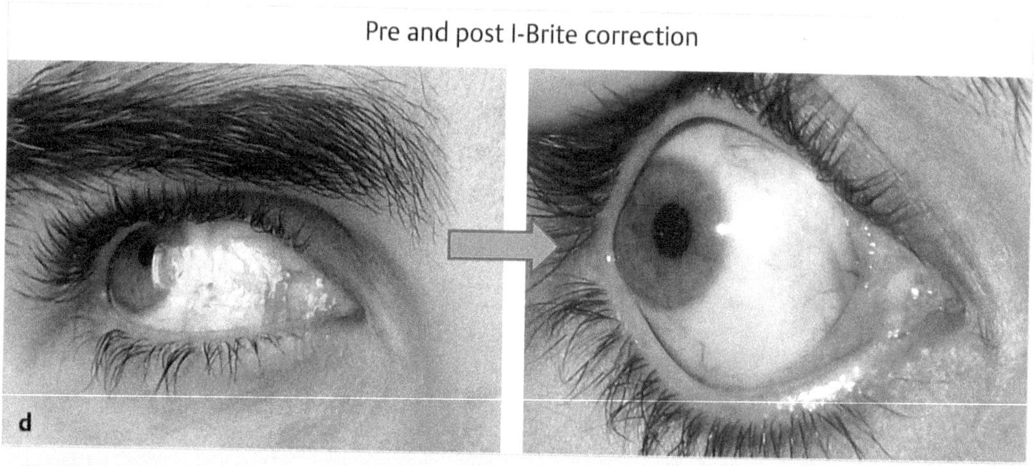

Pre and post I-Brite correction

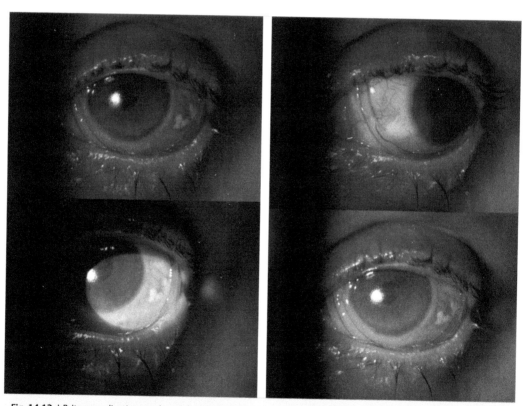

Fig. 14.11 (*continued*)

Fig. 14.12 I-Brite complications such as scleral calcific plaques can be controlled using ProKera technology to increase comfort while keeping surgery as backup if needed.

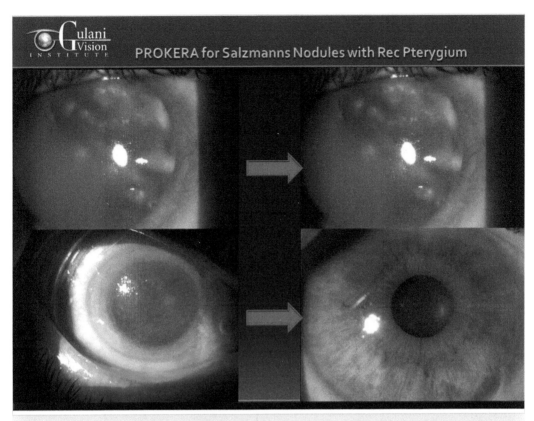

Fig. 14.13 Associated corneal scars and anterior corneal irregularities can be controlled with lamellar keratectomy and ProKera to a more stable surface for future vision correction.

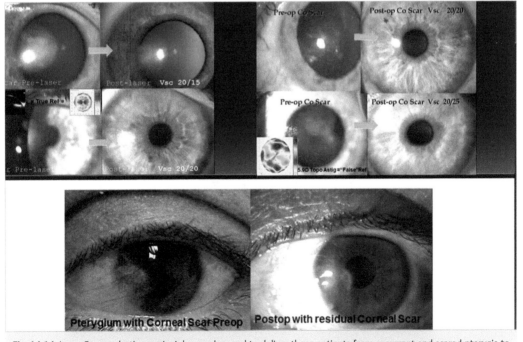

Fig. 14.14 Laser Corneoplastique principles can be used to deliver these patients from recurrent and scared pterygia to a staged refractive endpoint using excimer lasers.

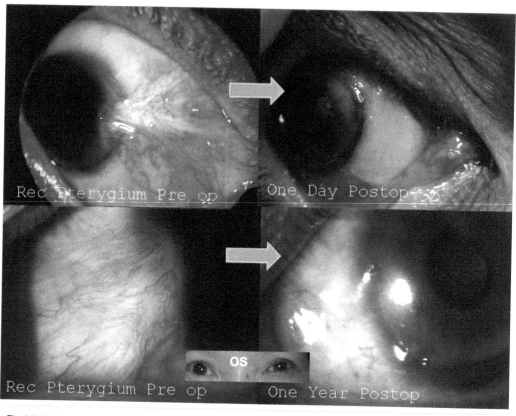

Fig. 14.15 Summary of recurrent and aggressive pterygia restored to cosmetic outcomes next day postoperative and long term. OS, oculus sinister.

complications and side effects empowers the surgeon to become a full-spectrum ocular surface surgeon who relentlessly follows the goals of raising the bar on ocular surface surgery to cosmetic outcomes in sync with enhancing vision simultaneously.

References

[1] Gulani AC. Sutureless amniotic surgery for pterygium: cosmetic outcomes for ocular surface surgery. Tech Ophthalmol. 2008; 6(2):41–44

[2] Gulani AC. No-stitch pterygium surgery: next day cosmetic outcomes. Video Journal of Ophthalmology 2009

[3] Gulani AC. Corneoplastique: art of vision surgery. Indian J Ophthalmol. 2014; 62(1):3–11

[4] Gulani A, Gulani A. Pterygium surgery: raising ocular surface surgery to cosmetic outcomes. Mastering Corneal Surgery: Recent Advances and Current Techniques. Thorofare, NJ: SLACK Incorporated; 2015:269–276 [chapter 25]

[5] Gulani AC. Gulani iceberg technique. Cataract & Refractive Surgery Today Europe. 2014; 9:48–49

[6] Gulani AC. A Cornea-friendly pterygium procedure. Rev Ophthalmol. 2012; 18(6):52–56

[7] Gulani A. Strategies for handling complex pterygium surgery, complications. Ophthamology Times. 2015; 40(7):11–17

[8] Gulani AC. Competencies in Oculoplastics: Anatomy, Trauma, Involutions, and Exam Preparation. New Retina MD. 2013:1–2

15 Pterygium and Pinguecula Surgery: Next-Day Cosmetic Outcomes

Arun C. Gulani and Aaishwariya A. Gulani

Abstract

Surgical correction of pterygium and pinguecula need to be raised to a cosmetic end point with least intervention, best vision, and aesthetic appearance. This along with enhanced safety and decreased recurrence rates will set the trend in raising the bar on ocular surface surgery itself.

Keywords: pinguecula surgery, pterygium surgery, Dr. Gulani Sparkle technique, no-stitch pterygium surgery, fibrin glue, amniotic graft, mitomycin C, cosmetic pterygium surgery

15.1 Introduction

Pterygium is one of the oldest pathologies known to ophthalmologists. Surgery for this condition can range from simple excision to techniques with exotic detail and meticulous maneuvers, with task-specific instruments beckoning an era of raised expectations and cosmetic outcomes in the field of ocular surface surgery itself.

For over nearly three decades, I have continued to hone my pterygium surgery technique and am convinced that it is the complete removal of pterygium/pinguecula—in particular, the surgical technique which is the crucial part for consistent success.[1,2,3]

Having performed practically every pterygium surgical technique and used nearly all kinds of graft material from autografts to allografts and synthetic variants including industry variants of the same, I conclusively made amniotic tissue[4,5,6] my choice grafting material for ocular surface reconstruction.

This choice was further underscored by Dr. Scheffer Tseng's travel to my surgical theater 16 years ago where he shared his body of work with amniotic tissue as I shared my desire to escalate this surgery to cosmetic outcomes very much like how Lasik surgery expectations had risen from 20/40 to 20/20.

May I encourage every eye surgeon to look at this surgery with that very mind-set. Once a surgeon has mastered the surgical technique, then and only then can they be assured of a consistent success pattern, which I shall be sharing in this chapter.

In summary, my protocol using the Iceberg surgical technique for pterygium involves a complete excision followed by mitomycin C application, which is then followed by a scaffold graft like amniotic tissue, with least traumatic healing incentives (sutureless/glue) resulting in consistent outcomes for patients from all over the world despite different heritage and cultures that encourage me to continue to offer and teach this surgical approach.

The part of the pterygium that is visible is only the tip of the iceberg (Iceberg concept). By removing only this visible portion, the main pathology with its tentacles is not addressed and remains hidden under the conjunctiva.

Though pterygia have been classified in many ways, most usually by the extent of involvement, my experience with varied presentations and outcomes in improving the surgical approach and outcomes over the years encouraged me to add an additional way to classify the pterygium based on the adhesion of the head locally, vascularity, and draw test for surrounding tissue involvement.

15.2 Head/Neck Adhesion

Peripheral/central adhesion can further be classified into diffuse, focal, and density based. In cases of peripheral adhesions, the pterygium easily peels off the cornea.

15.3 Vascularity

Engorged, tortous vessels, and simultaneous conjunctival fold contracture signify a more aggressive pterygium. This same concept can be used to determine outcomes postoperatively.

15.4 Draw Test

On tugging on the cornea, some pterygia may be small in size but outright gritty and deep into the cornea, resulting in thin cornea when removed. Preparation for this before surgery helps plan a smooth outcome (amniotic graft itself can be used as a lamellar fill). In addition, removal of these pterygia is more difficult from the corneal surface.

In the present series, we have used amniotic membrane, the innermost layer of the fetal membrane, for the treatment of pterygium wherein after the removal of proliferative tissue, amniotic membrane was placed on the sclera and adhered to the sclera with glue.

In my surgical approach, I continue to evolve my introduction of a nontraumatic, "no-stitch" technique using the criteria below and treat the pterygium as if it were a corneal scar (remember, with every surgery, I plan for unaided 20/20 and wish for surgery to leave the vision untouched or improved).

Thus, the basis of my surgical steps involves a lamellar corneal approach along with atraumatic yet complete pterygium removal as a conjunctival scar centripetally at the cornea and with full dissection right up to the roots, including all arising heads followed by subconjunctival mitomycin C application and amniotic graft layering on the sclera with glue and reconstructing the fornix in many cases. For simplicity of planning surgical approach and expectations including long-term impact, I have classified the criteria that allow me to custom design my surgery to each patient accordingly.

15.5 Surgical Criteria

- Extent of the pterygium.
- Density of the pterygium.
- Involvement of adjacent structures.
- Draw test.
- Head/neck adhesion.
- Vascularity.

The most common ocular surface pathologies that eye doctors see in their practice are pterygium and pinguecula.[7,8,9] These are intriguing pathologies that present themselves in various tissue distributions and vascular patterns. They can vary from small, atrophic lesions to large, aggressive fibrovascular growths that can, in advanced cases, compromise vision.

It is often suggested that prolonged exposure to the sun may instigate pterygia formation, and given anecdotal observations that it emerges more frequently among surfers and golf enthusiasts than in the general population (with greater prevalence in geographically predisposed areas), the relationship appears valid. I see patients from all over the world seeking the best cosmetic and functional outcome they can find. A decade ago, most patients seeking these services were predominantly models, TV news anchors, movie stars, and celebrities where looks were an integral part of their professional lifestyle. Recently, this trend has encompassed people from all walks of life, men and women alike. These patients present complaining that they are self-conscious about this condition, embarrassed by their appearance, and even depressed, in some cases.

In this chapter, I shall share my technique especially using glued, amniotic graft that I have used over nearly two decades on more than 600 eyes, with gratifying and consistent results (▶ Fig. 15.1, ▶ Fig. 15.2, ▶ Fig. 15.3). It enables not only those with cosmetic pterygia and pinguecula, but even those suffering from recurrent and aggressive vision-threatening pterygia, to expect clear, white eyes 1 day postoperatively. Starting with a sutured technique 20 years ago, and adding amniotic grafting 16 years ago, my method has since evolved into a sutureless procedure that incorporates the healing properties of human placenta. Patients are universally satisfied with their aesthetic results within 24 hours and are able to return to work and other daily activities within a couple of days.

This technique neither threatens nor adversely affects vision because there are no incisions involved in the cornea. While the average pterygium recurrence rate is commonly considered to hover around the 10 to 30% mark and higher, the recurrence rate with my technique is less than 0.5%.

My no-stitch technique utilizes human placenta as a scaffold bandage and chemical facilitator. It lends an elegant appearance to the eye and provides comfortable and expedited healing. My pterygia removal technique is called the "Gulani Iceberg Technique" because the part of the pterygium that is visible is just the tip of the iceberg, while the actual growth tends to be much deeper, and this surgical procedure addresses that.

15.6 Preparation to Surgery

In majority of cases, dry eye and ocular surface instability is an associated pathology and symptomatology (▶ Fig. 15.4 and ▶ Fig. 15.5). It is critical to take care of this not only for comfort, but also for long-term healing post pterygium surgery including anecdotally decreasing the progress of coexistent lesions, such as pinguecula in the same or contralateral eye.

Lacrimal plugs are an easy procedure that alleviates dry eye symptoms successfully in many

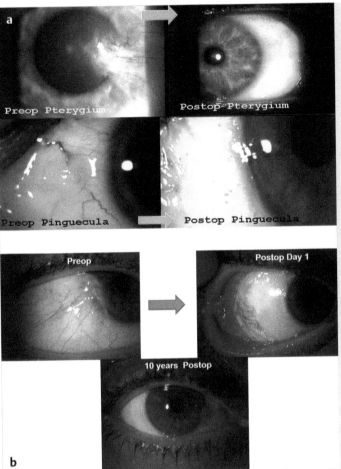

Fig. 15.1 (a) Preoperative pterygium. (b) Postoperative appearance day 1. (c) Pinguecula pre-op. (d) Pinguecula 1 day post-op.

aqueous-deficient cases. I usually select the lower lids to perform this procedure.

Meibomian gland dysfunction (MGD) is a commonly associated condition that can be addressed with ocular therapy including meibomian gland probing (MGP) using disposable probes (Rhein Medical, Tampa, FL) with topical anesthesia using a gel mixture made up of lidocaine and jojoba.

Having performed well over a 1,000 MGP procedures over the last 7 years, we have been extremely gratified with patient responses and satisfaction, not to mention an anecdotal improvement in postoperative surgical healing I have seen when clinically comparing my own postoperative care to that of 7 years ago, the surgical technique being the same.

Various technologies can be used for lid cleaning along with pharmaceutical adjuvants for lid and meibomian gland cleansing before or after accordingly.

Ocular surface stabilization before proceeding with pterygium surgery should be an integral function for a successful preoperative platform.

15.7 Step-by-Step Technique[10,11,12]

After a detailed informed consent and having planned my approach using the surgical criteria, my suture-free, three-step, pterygium and pinguecula removal technique includes mitomycin C, amniotic tissue, and Tisseel glue, to completion with patient's reaction next day in the mirror, observing the recently operated eye for appearance, comfort, and vision.

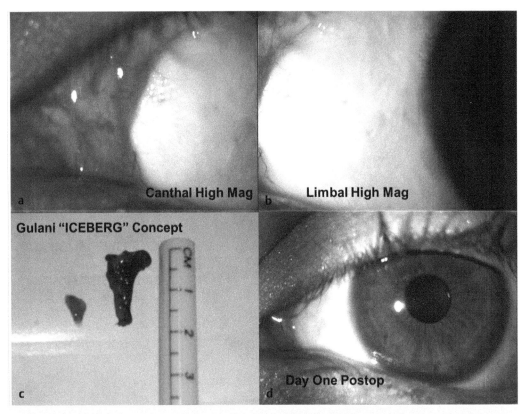

Fig. 15.2 (a) High magnification image of pterygium area at medial canthus (note cut end of remnant stump) post-op. (b) High magnification image of pterygium area at limbus post-op. (c) Iceberg concept: small lesion is clinically visible pterygium; the lesion next to it is the actual size on removal. (d) Same patient day 1 post-op with eye makeup.

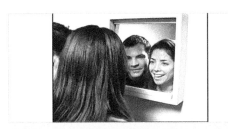

Fig. 15.3 Next day in the mirror: day 1 post surgery.

In a typical case, after topical anesthesia in the form of TetraVisc is applied with preoperative topical antibiotic drops, I begin with a fixation stitch at the opposite limbus using 7-o black silk and then mark the extent of the pterygium and visible interpalpebral area with a sterile marking pen. Intralesional anesthesia in the form of lidocaine with epinephrine is used (1–2 mL). (This can also delineate the extent of the pterygium in obscure

or recurrent cases.) Depending on the appearance and draw test, I will decide to approach the pterygium at the contracted medial conjunctival fold and proceed nasal to limbal (centripetal approach) or from the limbal head toward the medial conjunctival fold (centrifugal approach).

My mental attitude does not change whether the case is primary, recurrent, complex, or complicated (▶ Fig. 15.6, ▶ Fig. 15.7, ▶ Fig. 15.8, ▶ Fig. 15.9, ▶ Fig. 15.10, ▶ Fig. 15.11, ▶ Fig. 15.12, ▶ Fig. 15.13, ▶ Fig. 15.14, ▶ Fig. 15.15, ▶ Fig. 15.16, ▶ Fig. 15.17, ▶ Fig. 15.18). At the start of the procedure, the head of the pterygium is delineated from the cornea underneath. This can be done with posterior-to-anterior sweep using the Gulani pterygium cross-action spreader. In cases of mild adhesions, the pterygium can be easily separated from the cornea (mostly peripheral pterygia) or be effectively peeled in a single centrifugal movement.

The most important stage is dissecting the pterygium. The whole plane of the pterygium is

Ocular surface and tear film study

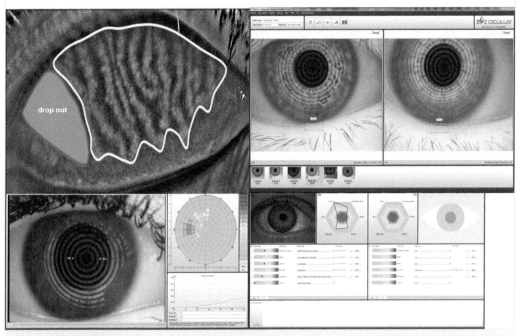

Fig. 15.4 and **15.5** Ocular surface analysis with tear film management along with meibomian gland dysfunction stabilization prior to surgery.

Meibomian gland disease (MGD)

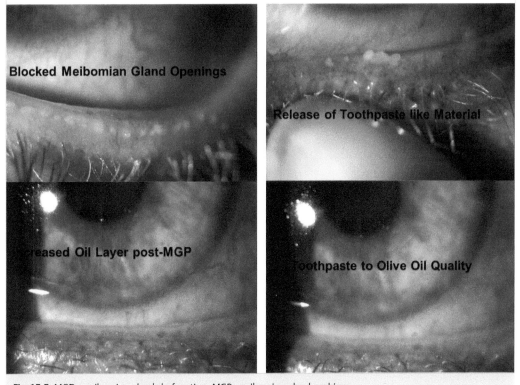

Fig. 15.5 MGD, meibomian gland dysfunction; MGP, meibomian gland probing.

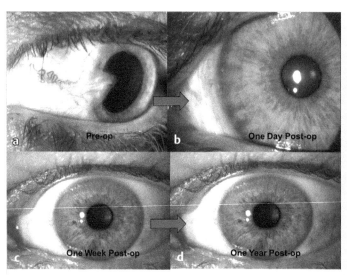

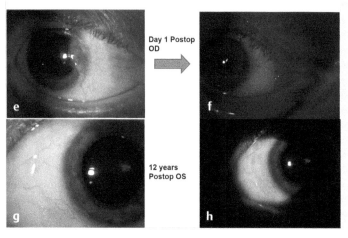

Fig. 15.6 (a) Central, focal, pterygium pre-op. (b) One day post-op. (c) One week post-op. (d) One year post-op. (e,f) 1 day post-op OD. (g,h) 12 years post-op OS. OD, oculus dexter; OS, oculus sinister.

delineated subconjunctivally as if separating a fan-shaped scar with tentacles into the fornices and medial angle. The pull is kept superior and vertical (to avoid damage to the underlying medial rectus). In cases of recurrent pterygium, I habitually use a modified muscle hook, Gulani muscle manipulator, to ascertain the anatomy by hooking the medial rectus. When the pterygium mass is removed, it resembles a spreading mass of tentacles. It is important to remove the entire mass to avoid recurrence, and the bleeding is usually minimal since there is actually no abrupt cutting, just separation with relieving tentacles.

The pterygium is dissected carefully superiorly, to avoid buttonholing the conjunctiva and invading the orbital septum, and inferiorly, to avoid cutting the underlying muscles, which is rechecked after the pterygium is removed.

A Weck-Cel sponge soaked in 1:1,000 epinephrine is used during this time tucked away into the nasal crevice where the cut pterygium stump is pressured into hemostasis. (In this way by the time this step is done, we approach a bloodless field again for dissection. Also, as added benefit, we have created space for tucking the future amniotic graft.)

After smoothing the cornea with a specially designed blunt blade, remnant tissue (especially in the gritty kind of pterygium) is meticulously removed with toothed forceps medial to limbal directions always. The blade is used again to smoothen the limbus.

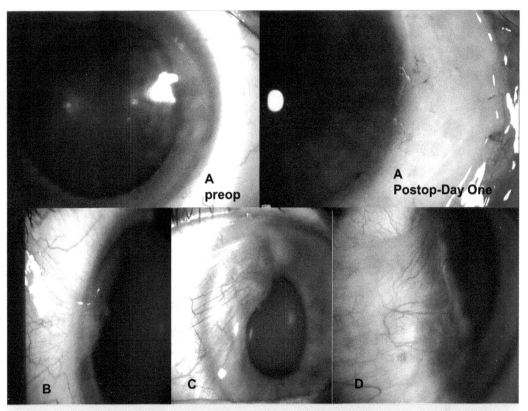

Fig. 15.7 (a) Central, diffuse, translucent pre-op. Next day post-op (b) peripheral and focal, (c) peripheral and diffuse, and (d) central, diffuse, and dense.

Aggressive pterygium: Day 1 post-op

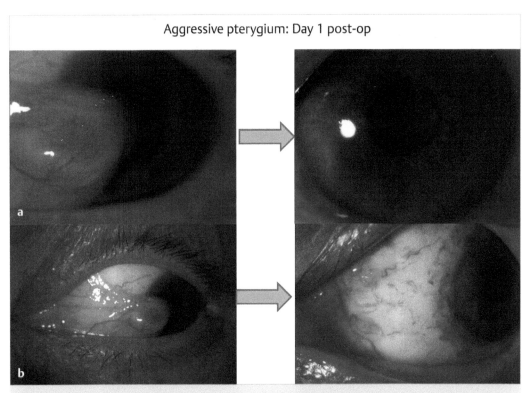

Fig. 15.8 (a,b) Aggressive medial impacting and raised bullous pterygium to cosmetic outcomes next day.

Gulani tissue grading
Site, extent, and density

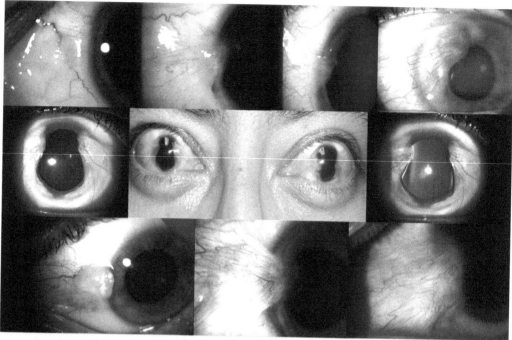

Fig. 15.9 Tissue grading system.

Gulani vascular grading
Tortuosity and density

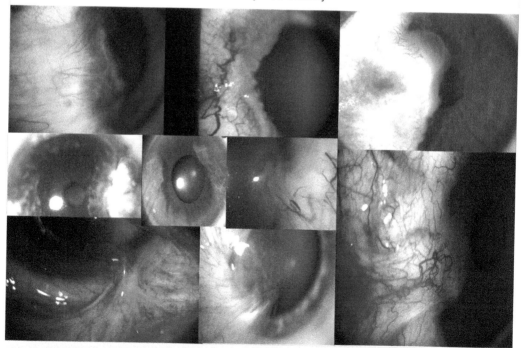

Fig. 15.10 Vascular grading system.

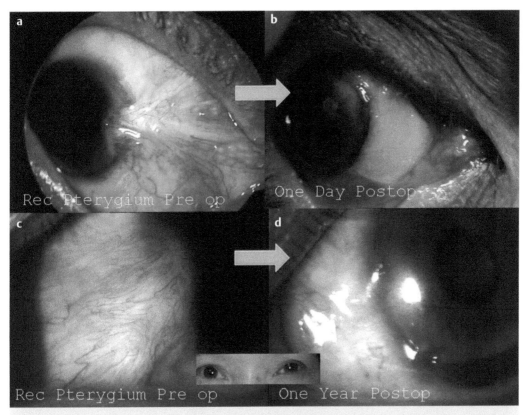

Fig. 15.11 (a) Recurrent, aggressive pterygium pre-op. (b) Day 1 postoperative appearance of same patient. (c) Multiple recurrent, aggressive pterygium pre-op. (d) One year postoperative appearance of the same patient.

There is none to very minimal bleeding during surgery. (The cautery is to be used sparingly and then only for cosmetic reasons.) Make it a point to patiently pick at the episcleral remnants to clear the underlying sclera in an attempt to remove all pterygium tissue from the area of impact.

Weck-Cel sponge pieces are soaked in mitomycin C 0.04%, placed under the conjunctiva (rolled over these pieces) in the area of the dissection, and are left in place for 30 seconds. Avoid application to sclera (in fact, dry the sclera with a clean Weck-Cel sponge). After removing the sponges to a full count, the area is flushed with copious balanced salt solution.

I will then receive the amniotic graft onto the cornea which acts like an illuminated "receiving table" (since by now the retroillumination from pupillary dilation from local epinephrine that was used along with the Weck-Cel for hemostasis provides an elegant glow), slide it onto the bare sclera, and sweep it into place under the medial, superior,

and inferior conjunctiva using what I call a no-touch "tyre–tool" technique. Next, I will use two separate syringes to deliver each component of the Tisseel glue beneath the amniotic graft in a controlled fashion. I now use a Weck-Cel sponge to squeegee the graft on the sclera and also to swipe the fornices for any excess glue to avoid the possibility of postoperative keratitis/foreign body sensation. Then I use the same no. 64 blade in a single, controlled motion to trim the excess amniotic graft along the limbus using a single circumlinear motion. The cut is deep enough to cut the amniotic graft, but not the cornea. I will then peel away the excessive amniotic tissue to facilitate an elegant outcome; these patients can wear contact lenses the next day or get ready for refractive surgery soon after. In many cases of corneal involvement, I also plan for self-retaining amniotic membrane graft in bandage contact lens placement next day postoperatively. We have had no graft slippage in our series of patients and have had consistent,

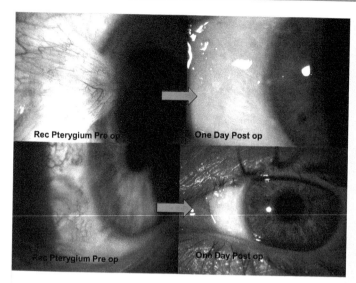

Fig. 15.12 (a) Recurrent, aggressive pterygium pre-op. (b) Day 1 postoperative appearance of same patient. (c) Multiple recurrent, aggressive pterygium pre-op. (d) One year postoperative appearance of the same patient.

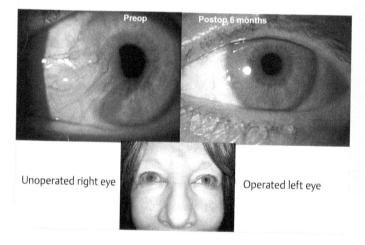

successful long-term outcomes 1-day postoperatively among patients regardless of age, sex, or race.

The postoperative regimen comprises steroid drops four times a day for the first week and then tapered down every week by one drop for 1 month. Nonsteroidal drops are prescribed two times a day for 2 weeks, and antibiotic drops are prescribed four times a day for 2 weeks.

Since many patients seeking this surgery are healthy and are in their youth, they have opted for laryngeal mask airway (LMA) as an anesthesia option, and I am fine with that, having conferred with our anesthesiologist over nearly a decade

regarding safety and also comfort given the extensive dissection technique.

15.8 Side Effects and Complications

Despite the consistency of our results and a satisfied worldwide clientele, I am very careful to emphasize to all my patients that even though their complaints are often of a cosmetic nature, this is a surgical procedure, and as with any surgical procedure, there are associated risks. Even with a recurrence rate of less than 0.5%, the risk of

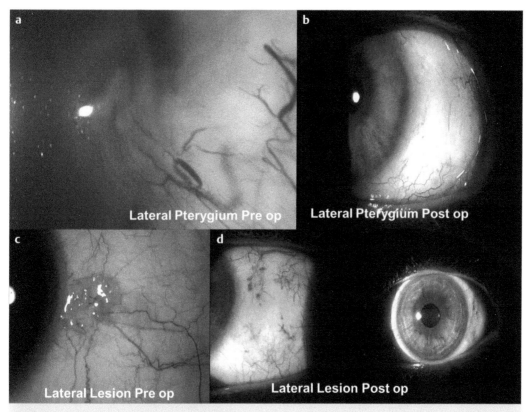

Fig. 15.13 (a-d) Lateral pterygium pre and post-op.

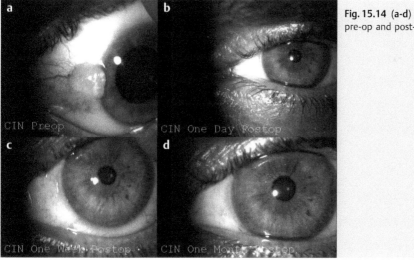

Fig. 15.14 (a-d) Carcinoma in situ pre-op and post-op.

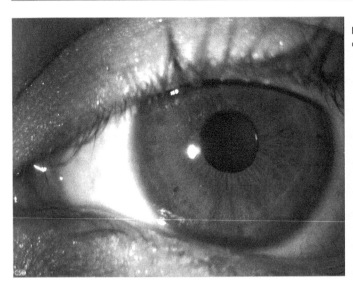

Fig. 15.15 Grade 1 appearance next day post-op pterygium surgery.

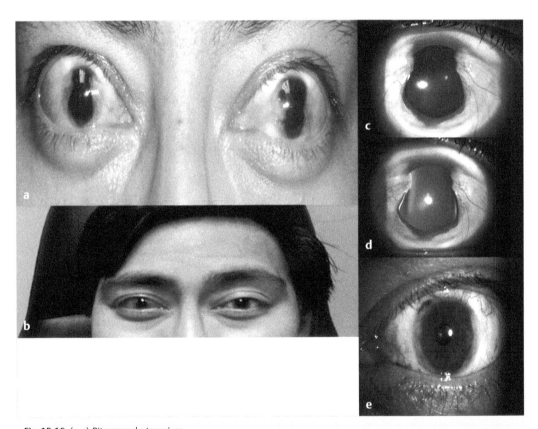

Fig. 15.16 (a-e) Bitemporal pterygium.

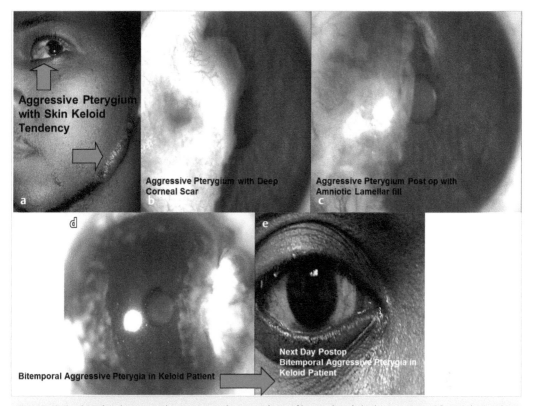

Fig. 15.17 (a-e) High-risk cases with systemic and extraocular profiles, such as keloids. Amniotic grafts can be used in such cases as an extension of lamellar fill, which gradually resolves over time and can be followed up by laser vision surgery.

untoward effects, including scarring and the possibility of a worse looking eye, remains.

I do not support luring advertisements, deals, or gimmicks and surely do not promise that this is a trivial procedure.

Every patient must verbalize full understanding of this surgery and possible impact on their lives including long-term effects, and after confirmation of the same, I accept to do their surgery.

I have seen self-corrected side effects and outcomes like subamniotic blood (▶ Fig. 15.19 and ▶ Fig. 15.20) in a postoperative patient with accidental trauma resolved over a week, which cleared in a month, while a case of scleral thinning resolved on artificial tears over 3 months.

Of five cases of pyogenic granulomas postoperatively, three resolved on topical steroids, while two required cautery excision for excellent long-term healing and appearance with no recurrence.

Three cases with adverse circumstances in my experience that are etched on my soul include a patient who was perfectly satisfied with a sparkling white eye after surgery. When he flew back home, his eye surgeon did not see any stitches or red areas postoperatively, so the surgeon rubbed a Q-tip across the eye and rubbed the glued graft off the eye. This patient flew back to me and needed regrafting. In another case, a patient needed muscle alignment surgery, and in another instance, a patient is being followed up for a localized pupil-shape anomaly that is improving. All three of these cases were of extensive bitemporal surgery; hence, I continue to recommend that patients have only one lesion removed at a time.

I continue to collect information and postoperative data on my surgical patients who fly back to their surgeons in different states or countries to keep reporting outcomes and make sure that my integrity is a backbone to my desire in propelling cosmetic outcomes for pterygium surgery.

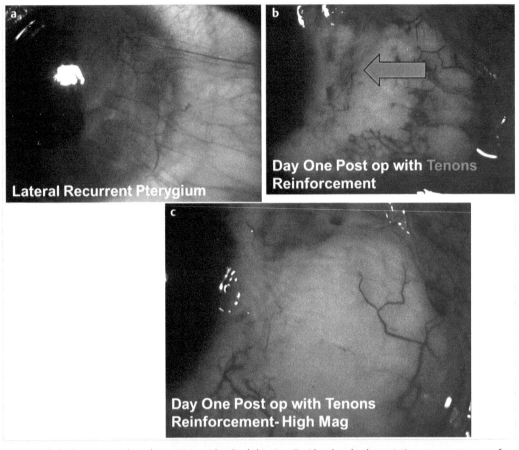

Fig. 15.18 (a-c) Aggressive lateral pterygium with scleral thinning. Besides the glued, amniotic surgery, a tongue of adjacent tenons (arrow) was used to cover the thin area after stacking amniotic graft tissue.

15.9 Recurrent Pterygia

I again want to emphasize, the "MINDSET." Do not worry about who operated and in which state and country; believe that this patient can have a sparkling eye and the surgery is really not difficult.

Being a referral center for pterygium and pinguecula complication surgeries from surgeons worldwide, I have seen many presentations and patient outcomes that ranged from mildly disturbing to devastating. Just like everything else, manage the patient expectations and perform with your best intention to a flawless goal.

In fact, I approach these cases exactly as I would approach virgin pterygium cases; only in many such cases, I can see the residual pterygium that the previous surgeon had left behind. The surgery is exactly the same no matter how aggressive and recurrent the pterygium is. The bleeding is again

very minimal if you follow these pearls in recurrent cases, that is, select an area which is more amenable to approach and dissect down into this area until you reach the scleral bed (most usually the previous ophthalmologist must have done a meticulous job of clearing the sclera). Once you reach sclera, dissect from behind forward and the whole pterygium mass will lift up in a form I call the "Armor Technique" (very much like a thick plate of armor).

Once again, bleeding will be minimal (avoid the tendency to cut and vigorously dissect; that will lead to bleeding and losing the plane of easy dissection). Follow through with mitomycin C and amniotic tissue with glue as mentioned and take care of any associated pathologies such as fornix reconstruction, corneal scar management, and reinforcing associated thinned out sclera if needed.

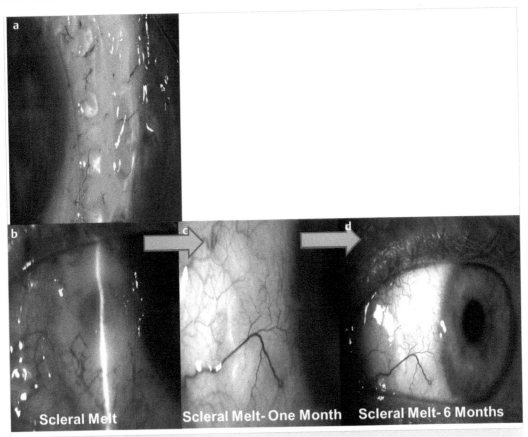

Fig. 15.19 (a–d) Self-limiting adverse events: amniotic "bubble wrap" sign. Self-resolving scleral melt, which resolved over 1 to 3 months.

15.10 Pinguecula Surgery

Pterygium surgery has led itself to an increase in the requests for pinguecula removal for patients in whom their appearance may be troubling to the patient or threatens their livelihood itself (models, TV news anchors, sales personnel, etc.).

Having interviewed patients who fly to me from all over the world, I found that they are affected by their pingueculae and described their feelings ranging from "self-conscious" to "low self-esteem" and even "depression" in some cases, thus making it an important item to address in their eye examinations with their eye doctors who usually disregard pingueculae complaints as trivial.

I teach this as a similar request we used to get nearly two decades ago when our Lasik results for high ammetropia were confidently predictable enough that we realized patients seeking correction of low refractive errors deserved our attention.

Here again, since the bar has been raised on outcomes, pinguecula removal follows the same principle as pterygium surgery only with a higher level of responsibility since a less than perfect outcome will look like a relative complication given the starting point was not so bad to begin with.

Pinguecula requests started in my practice with models, movie stars, and celebrities, mostly female, and now are nearly equal in demand with males and by patients from all walks of life.

15.11 Next Day Postoperative: "In the Mirror" Protocol

Two decades ago, I wanted to raise the bar for pterygium surgery similar to the expectations from Lasik surgery, where the outcomes, no matter how aggressive or complicated, of pterygia would be a flawless appearance starting next day and with a safety backing for the rest of their lives. I

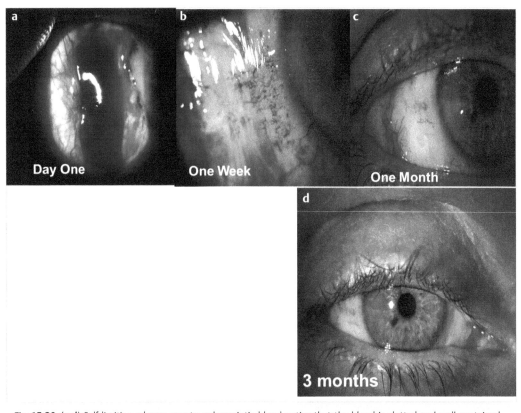

Fig. 15.20 (**a-d**) Self-limiting adverse events: subamniotic blood notice that the blood is clotted and well contained under the amniotic graft limited by the glued rectangular boundary of the graft and self-resolution is noted.

Table 15.1 Objective grading of the postoperative site on the basis of external and slit-lamp examination

Gulani objective grading	Examination findings on the postoperative site
Grade 1	Better than normal appearance of operative site (pearly white)
Grade 2	Normal appearance of the eye and scleral area
Grade 3	Presence of fine episcleral vessels in the excised Area.
Grade 4	Episcleral vessels reaching the limbus
Grade 5	Fibrovascular tissue in the excised area reaching to the limbus
Grade 6	Fibrovascular tissue invading the cornea
Grade 7	Worse than preoperative appearance
Grade 8	Symblepharon and restrictive eye movements in addition to Grade 7

have held myself accountable in making patients walk up to the mirror next day to look and exclaim whatever they feel like. Besides this subjective response, we also document an objective assessment on day 1 postoperatively (▶ Table 15.1, ▶ Table 15.2, ▶ Table 15.3, ▶ Table 15.4, ▶ Table 15.5).

You can see that many of the patients especially the Type A personalities will even wear make-up next day despite our restricting them preoperatively.

This cosmetic appeal of the outcome with the no-stitch, no-patch, and no-red approach along with absence of visual deficit is raising the bar in patients now seeking this approach for related ocular surface conditions, such as pinguecula and conjunctivochalasis.

Table 15.2 Grading of the amniotic graft placement post operatively on day 1

Gulani objective grading of the postoperative amniotic graft area	Examination findings on the amniotic graft area
Grade 1	Clear with good placement
Grade 2	Good placement but with bubble-wrap appearance
Grade 3	Displaced graft
Grade 4	Subamniotic blood

Table 15.3 Postoperative grading of the cornea on the basis of slit-lamp examination

Gulani objective grading of the postoperative cornea	Examination findings of the postoperative cornea
Grade 1	Clear
Grade 2	Mild keratitis
Grade 3	Clouding at surgical site
Grade 4	Lamellar fill

Table 15.4 Subjective grading of postoperative appearance day 1 (slide 25)

Gulani day 1 post-op patient subjective response scale	Appearance
Grade 1	Cannot tell which eye had surgery
Grade 2	Can tell which eye had surgery, but looks untouched
Grade 3	Operated eye looks red, but acceptable
Grade 4	Operated eye looks beefy red and unacceptable

Note: Subjective grading: The day after the procedure, patients walked up to a mirror, examined the operative site, and gave a verbal subjective exclamation, which was documented as the postoperative patient subjective assessment of appearance. The verbal subjective response was graded on a scale of 1 to 4. This exclamation was based on the flawless, clear appearance of the operated eye with equal lid openings. Subjective responses recorded the day after the procedure to measure patient discomfort upon eye movements was also recorded and titled patient subjective assessment of symptoms and was graded on a scale of 1 to 3.

Table 15.5 Subjective grading of discomfort day 1 postoperative

Gulani day 1 post-op patient subjective symptom scale	Level of discomfort
Grade 1	No discomfort
Grade 2	Some discomfort
Grade 3	Uncomfortable

15.12 Look Good, See Good!

As I always teach, no eye surgery is complete without addressing the patient's vision.[13,14,15] It is our duty and responsibility to make sure that we do not compromise vision in any form at all with this surgery.

Besides aiming for a normal-looking eye, I strive to maintain their vision status (in some cases, patients may have had Lasik surgery, etc., or in many cases, they can now become candidates for Lasik or premium cataract surgery [▶ Fig. 15.21, ▶ Fig. 15.22, ▶ Fig. 15.23, ▶ Fig. 15.24, ▶ Fig. 15.25, ▶ Fig. 15.26, ▶ Fig. 15.27] once we clear the cornea and stabilize the ocular surface).

Additionally, one can stage corneal scar surgery following pterygium surgery to emmetropia—Corneoplastique.

We shall discuss more about this topic in our next chapter.

In my practice, which has a referral base of patients from all over the world, I have had the privilege to evaluate and operate on an extensive variety of patients with pterygium and pinguecula presentations, and with our ongoing experience, it is our pleasure to report on these outcomes. We are publishing our series of 600 cases of pterygium surgery using the above-mentioned technique with less than 0.5% recurrence and also extent of follow-up for cases up to 16 years postoperatively.

In summary, pterygium and pinguecula surgery outcomes (the very next day postoperative) with safety and long-term stability (▶ Fig. 15.28, ▶ Fig. 15.29, ▶ Fig. 15.30, ▶ Fig. 15.31) with methods described above have made my dream of aesthetic outcomes for ocular surface a reality. May I encourage you to have this mindset and pursue these goals.

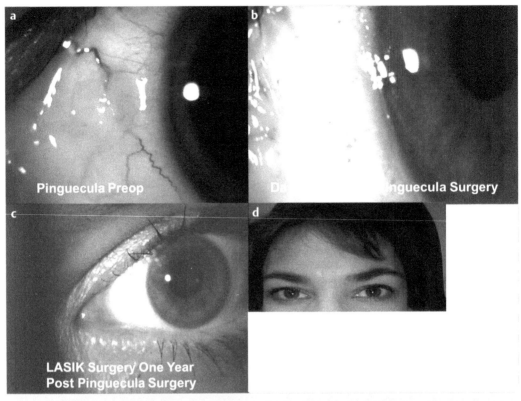

Fig. 15.21 (a-d) Pinguecula pre- and post-op followed by Lasik surgery for vision correction. Laser vision surgery can be commenced early due to excellent and rapid healing to avail patients of vision besides aesthetic outcomes.

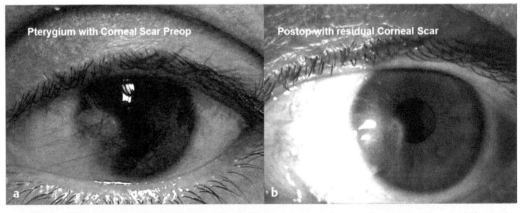

Fig. 15.22 (a,b) Residual corneal scar, which is embedded in the cornea, can be seen after successful removal of central, aggressive, visual axis impacting pterygium.

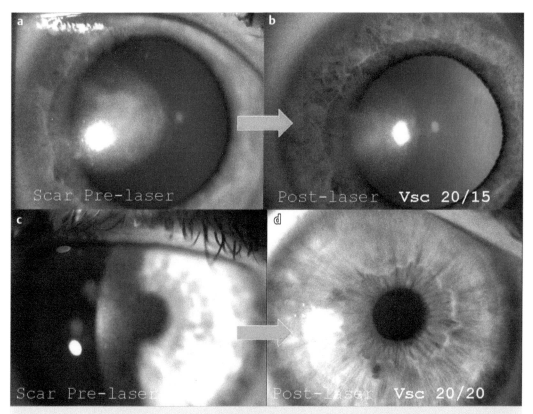

Fig. 15.23 (a-d) Residual scars corrected to emmetropia using the excimer laser following Corneoplastique™ principles.

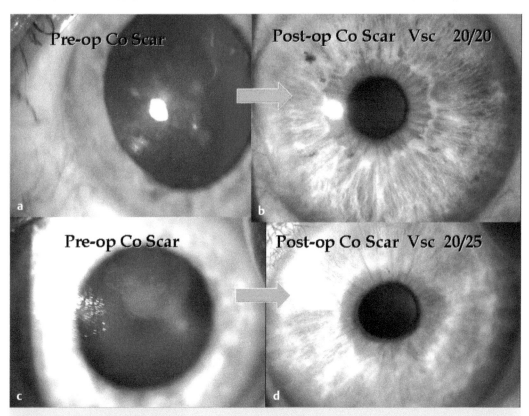

Fig. 15.24 (a-d) Overlying corneal scars can be peeled off the cornea and refractive laser surgery can be performed following Corneoplastique™ principles.

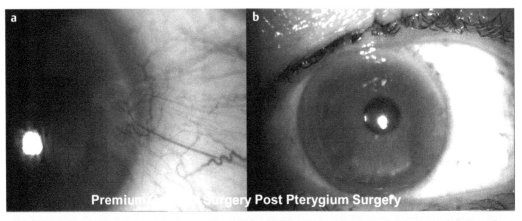

Premium **gery Post Pterygium Surgery**

Fig. 15.25 (a,b) Premium cataract surgery can be performed following pterygium surgery once corneal clarity and measurability along with stability has been attained.

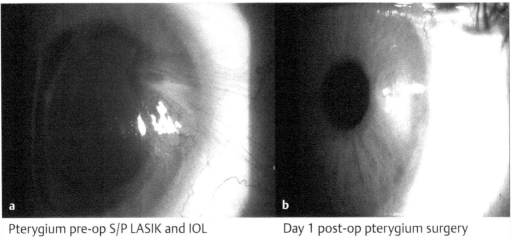

Pterygium pre-op S/P LASIK and IOL

Day 1 post-op pterygium surgery
S/P LASIK and IOL

Fig. 15.26 (a,b) Patients with previous Lasik and or premium cataract surgery can undergo pterygium surgery making sure that there are no incisions on the cornea as such patients will not tolerate a drop in their vision (20/20 pre-op, 20/20 post-op).

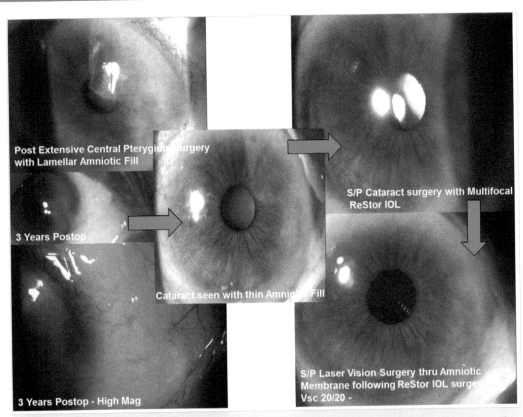

Post Extensive Central Pterygium Surgery with Lamellar Amniotic Fill

3 Years Postop

Cataract seen with thin Amniotic Fill

3 Years Postop - High Mag

S/P Cataract surgery with Multifocal ReStor IOL

S/P Laser Vision Surgery thru Amniotic Membrane following ReStor IOL surgery Vsc 20/20 -

Fig. 15.27 A patient who underwent pterygium surgery 3 years ago. She had a very aggressive pterygium covering the visual axis of the cornea. This area was covered as a lamellar fill with extended amniotic graft, which can be seen as a flap of translucent tissue. She underwent cataract surgery with multifocal lens implant (ReStor) in a planned, staged process followed by laser surgery through her amniotic graft to correct the corneal surface and refractive error to excellent unaided vision. IOL, intraocular lens. S/P, status post; Vsc, uncorrected visual acuity.

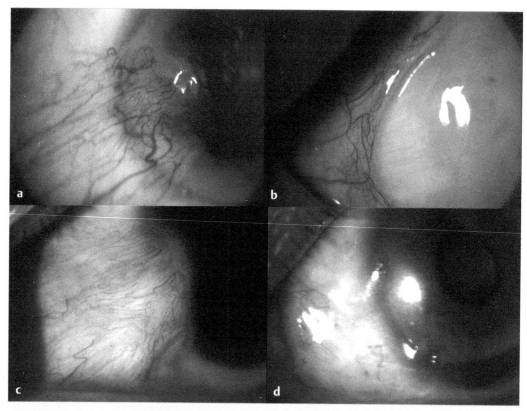

Fig. 15.28 (a-d) Aggressive, high vascular or tissue-graded pterygia should still experience the same next day cosmetic outcomes.

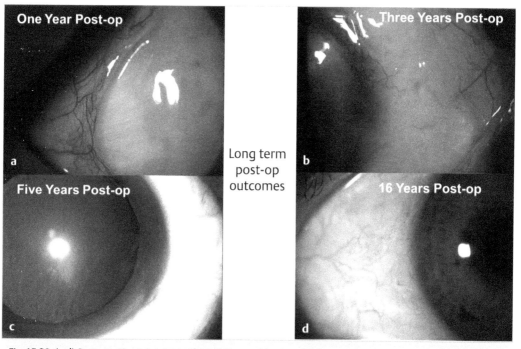

Fig. 15.29 (a-d) Postoperative appearances from 1 to over 16 years of follow-up.

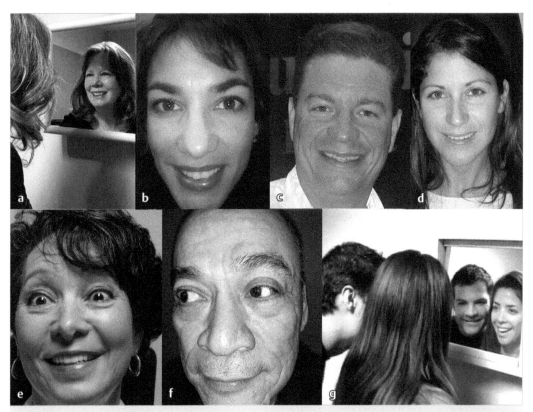

Fig. 15.30 (a-g) Day 1 post-op faces of the pterygium surgery patients (of all ages, sex, and race), including looking into the mirror on day 1 post-op.

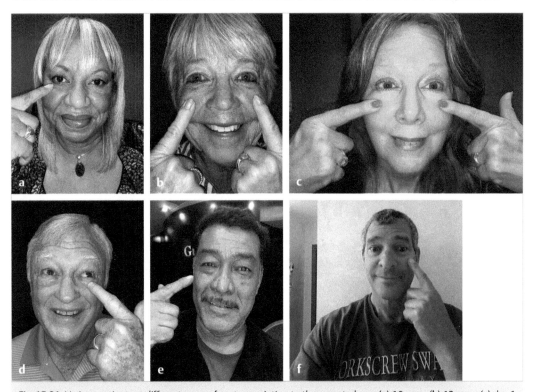

Fig. 15.31 Various patients at different years of post op pointing to the operated eye. (a) 16 years (b) 12 years (c) day 1 (d) 10 years (e) 14 years (f) 14 years.

15.13 Acknowledgements

I would like to thank Aaishwariya A. Gulani (Wharton School of Business, University of Pennsylvania), Research Coordinator: Gulani Vision Institute.

References

[1] Gulani A, Dastur YK. Simultaneous pterygium and cataract surgery. J Postgrad Med. 1995; 41(1):8–11

[2] Gulani AC. Sutureless amniotic surgery for pterygium: cosmetic outcomes for ocular surface surgery. Tech Ophthalmol. 2008; 6(2):41–44

[3] Gulani AC. A cornea-friendly pterygium procedure. Rev Ophthalmol. 2012; 18(6):52–56

[4] Trelford JD, Trelford-Sauder M. The amnion in surgery, past and present. Am J Obstet Gynecol. 1979; 134(7):833–845

[5] Tayyar M, Turan R, Ayata D. The use of amniotic membrane plus heparin to prevent postoperative adhesions in the rabbit. Tokai J Exp Clin Med. 1993; 18(1–2):57–60

[6] Kim JC, Tseng SCG. Transplantation of preserved human amniotic membrane for surface reconstruction in severely damaged rabbit corneas. Cornea. 1995; 14(5):473–484

[7] Coroneo MT, Di Girolamo N, Wakefield D. The pathogenesis of pterygia. Curr Opin Ophthalmol. 1999; 10(4):282–288

[8] Elliott R. The aetiology of pterygium. Trans Ophthalmol Soc N Z. 1961; 13 Suppl:22–41

[9] Blum HF. Carcinogenesis by Ultraviolet Light. Princeton, NJ: Princeton University Press; 1959

[10] Gulani AC. Gulani iceberg technique. Cataract Refrac Surg Today Europe.. 2014; 9:48–49

[11] Gulani A. Raising the bar on pterygium and pinguecula surgery. Ophthalmology Times. 2015; 40(6):24–30

[12] Gulani A, Gulani A. Pterygium surgery rising ocular surface surgery to cosmetic outcomes. In: Mastering Corneal Surgery: Recent Advances and Current Techniques. Thorofare: SLACK Incorporated, 2015:25–29

[13] Gulani AC. "Corneoplastique™": Art of Ocular Surface and Refractive Surgery. South African Refractive & Cataract Surgery Proceedings. August 2005

[14] Gulani AC. Surgical method sets higher standard for managing pterygium. Ocular Surgery News. Consultation Section, August 2008

[15] Gulani AC. Pterygium and pinguecula surgery: cosmetic desires for future of ocular surface surgery. Video Journal of Ophthalmology; 2009

16 Kerato-Refractive and Premium Cataract Surgery with Pterygium

Arun C. Gulani and Aaishwariya A. Gulani

Abstract

Cosmetic surgical outcomes of pterygium and pinguecula have allowed many patients previously considered "not a candidate" to candidacy for Lasik, premium cataract surgery, and a wide spectrum of kerato-lenticulo-refractive techniques to enable patients with ocular surface disorder to see and to look great.

Keywords: Lasik, femto second laser, cataract surgery, premium cataract surgery, multifocal lens implants, kerato-refractive surgery, not a candidate, no-stitch pterygium surgery, Corneoplastique

16.1 Introduction

Having mastered the art of performing pterygium and pinguecula surgery to a cosmetic outcome with minimal refractive inducement on the cornea leads us to offer premium cataract and laser vision surgery to these patients who otherwise were relegated to the category of "not a candidate" (▶ Fig. 16.1, ▶ Fig. 16.2).

On the other end of this spectrum are cases of successful Lasik and premium cataract surgery who may have developed subsequent pterygium or pinguecula surgery, and it is our responsibility to maintain or enhance that good vision is achieved while operating on their ocular surface.

These two goals at the end of a large spectrum highlight my desire to conquer and share the final frontier in ocular surface surgery: Look Good, See Good!

So, let us first understand the gravity of this situation and need for recognition enough to make us visually accountable while performing ocular surface surgery including pterygium surgery.

Even if my practice has a global referral base of complex cases, I am sure in most practices, pterygium or pinguecula patients usually present with associated ammetropia be it myopia, hyperopia, or astigmatism and of course, presbyopia in some cases.

Many of these patients cannot wear contact lenses comfortably due to irregular eye globe contour caused by existent pterygium mass or irregular corneal contour due to associated corneal involvement by pterygium or scars.

Additionally, even if some of them fit well, most of these cases have ocular surface instability and dry eyes, which make their contact lens wearing an uncomfortable experience even with a good fit.

Also, since millions of patients worldwide have undergone vision corrective surgery as Lasik or cataract surgery, we must honor the vision that their previous surgeon had delivered for them,[1,2] and thus be very conscious in our pterygium surgery dissection to avoid any refractive error inducement.

I have stratified the impact of pterygium on vision and refractive surgery into the following anatomically related categories:

16.2 Ocular Surface

- Tear film instability and deficiency
- Bulk effect in distorting globe contour

16.3 Conjunctival

- Bulk effect in distorting globe contour
- Forniceal distortion and irregular conjunctival distortion thus making it difficult for suction based technology, i.e., Lasik, INTACS, and femtosecond cataract surgery

16.4 Corneal

- Scar, which affects vision directly
- Irregular ammetropia (most usually astigmatism)
- Higher order aberrations
- Inaccurate refractive and keratometry measurements, thus impacting accurate Laser vision or cataract surgery

In summary, all of the above categories need to be normalized and made accurately measureable to proceed with any vision corrective surgery.

You can see now how performing pterygium surgery or pinguecula surgery, or for that matter, any ocular surface surgery becomes an intense

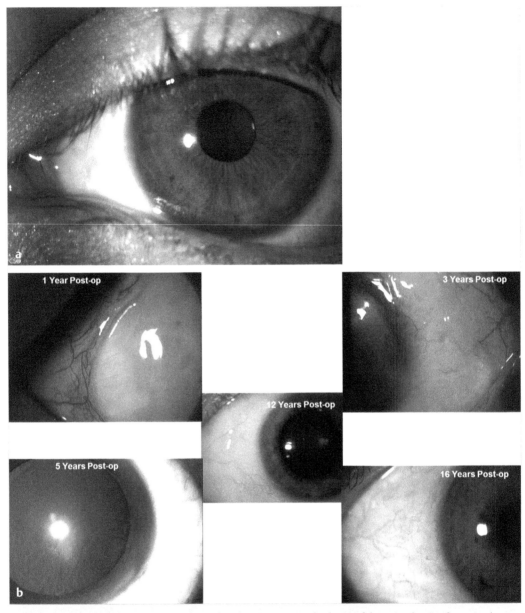

Fig. 16.1 (a,b) Next-day cosmetic outcomes and 16 years' experience lead to confidence in planning for a visual platform besides aiming for cosmetic appearance. Postop, postoperatively.

technique where you have to worry about vision, to either maintain or enhance it with your surgery while aspiring for a cosmetic outcome.

For the sake of simplifying this full-spectrum pterygium surgical allocations,[3,4] I have divided them into two basic categories to aid kerato-lenticulo-refractive endeavors:

1. Prepare the cornea and ocular surface.
2. Repair the cornea and ocular surface.

These two categories will summarize majority of the cases we see in our everyday practice with a desire to either take every patient to cosmetic outcomes and also provide options for premium

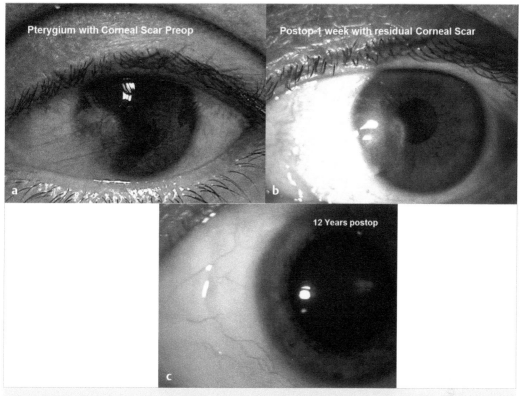

Fig. 16.2 (a-c) Aggressive pterygium with scar with clearance and stability at 12 years postop.

refractive surgery or at least, maintain their best vision if they have had refractive surgery in the past.

As I always teach, no eye surgery is complete without addressing the patient's vision. For instance, the elegance of this no-stitch amniotic graft technique enables many patients who were initially non-candidates for laser refractive surgery or premium lens refractive surgery (due to tissue-induced irregular astigmatism, corneal scars, tear film instability, or higher order aberrations) to be safely prepared for vision corrective surgery, such as Lasik, laser surface ablation, and even premium IOL (intraocular lens implant) cataract surgery. The removal of corneal scars and pterygium tissue, and the resultant clear and measurable optical system, in essence safely and elegantly convert patients from non-refractive surgery candidates into refractive surgery candidates. Given the active lifestyles of patients of all age groups today along with their demands for cosmetic appeal and vision freedom we can therefore plan vision corrective surgery fowling a foundation of successful ocular surface surgery (▶ Fig. 16.3).

Also, given that many patients who present with pterygium and pinguecula have already had some form of laser vision surgery or premium lens surgery, this provides a method to maintain their optimized vision during pterygium surgery because it does not distort Lasik flaps, induce, or cause corneal desiccation/distortion with traumatic techniques or refractively adverse corneal incisions.

So, in my practice, these patients will undergo laser vision surgery and/or premium cataract surgery in not so distant succession since the cornea is basically cleared (for laser ASA) with excellent globe contour or for the suction ring during Lasik and even INTACS or femtosecond laser application in premium cataract surgery; the concept of *Look Good, See Good*!

I have performed Lasik, laser PRK surface ablation, premium cataract surgery using multifocal and toric lens implants, astigmatic keratotomy, phakic implants in high myopia, and even INTACS microsegments for keratoconus in patients who have undergone my amniotic graft pterygium and pinguecula removal surgery with successful

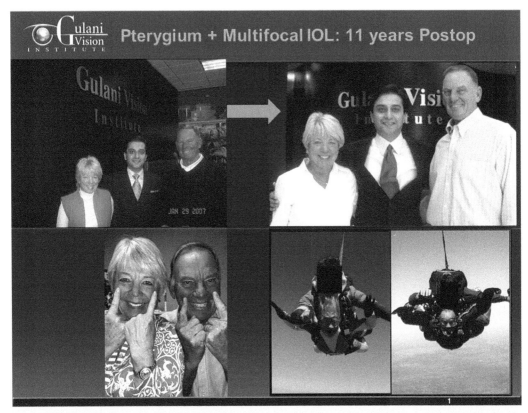

Fig. 16.3 We see this active couple who underwent my pterygium surgery to a cosmetic outcome which also simultaneously restored their corneal irregularity to a smooth measurable refraction so we could confidently then allow them to elect for Premium Cataract surgery with Multifocal Lens implants to 20/20 vision at all distances without glasses. At 11 years postoperative gate they are still enjoying sparkling white eyes with 20/20 vision without any glasses and actively pursuing life's many sporty endeavors.

outcomes. Given the no-cut nature of this ocular surface procedure, there is no induced refractive change with this technique—thereby maintaining good vision or perhaps even improving vision by relieving the astigmatism caused by pterygium-induced pull on the cornea.

It is our responsibility to ensure that we are not jeopardizing vision in any form and in fact provide options for vision correction using modalities mentioned above, such as Lasik, PRK, cataract surgery,[5] INTACS, etc. using Corneoplastique principles for an early visual rehabilitation of the operated eye. Given that numerous patients have undergone Lasik and cataract surgery all over the world, we are seeing patients who need surgery for pterygium/pinguecula after these vision correcting surgeries. Here, it is vital not to affect the vision in any way, as these patients shall not tolerate a drop in their excellent 20/20 outcomes.

Having raised this concept further, I have planned a staged process in many aggressive cases to first remove the pterygium followed by laser Corneoplastique to address the associated "On-Cornea" or "In-Cornea" scars straight to 20/20 (▶ Fig. 16.4a, b–▶ Fig. 16.5a-c).

In "On-Cornea" scars, we need to peel these scars and apply the excimer laser in a refractive mode not relying on the "Clown-suit" corneal topography with its false appearance of high irregular astigmatism. In the "In-Cornea" scars, we follow their refraction and corneal topography straight to 20/20 using refractive excimer laser application.[6]

Thus, clearing the cornea and making it more accurately measurable while also improving the eye globe surface regularity allow to approach these patients like a normal refractive surgery candidate and deliver vision without glasses or contact lenses.

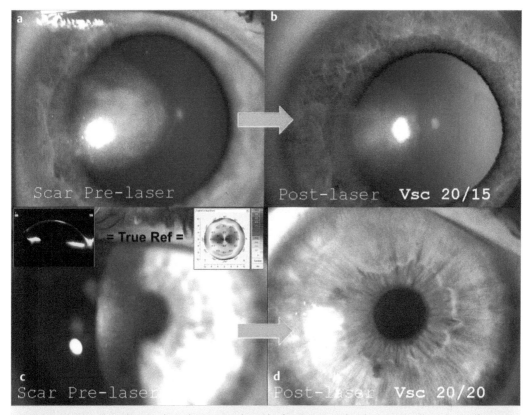

Fig. 16.4 (a-e) "In-Corneal" scar where the topography and refraction are real and can proceed with laser refractive Surgery to clearance and emmetropic vision. Vsc, unaided visual acuity. (*continued*)

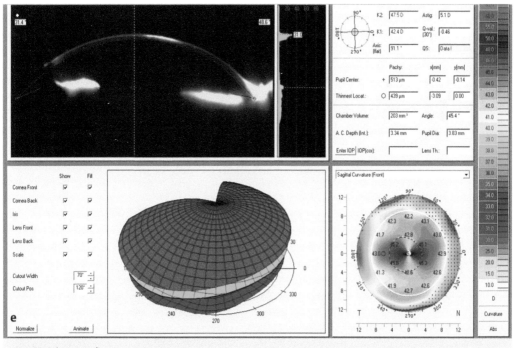

Fig. 16.4 (*continued*)

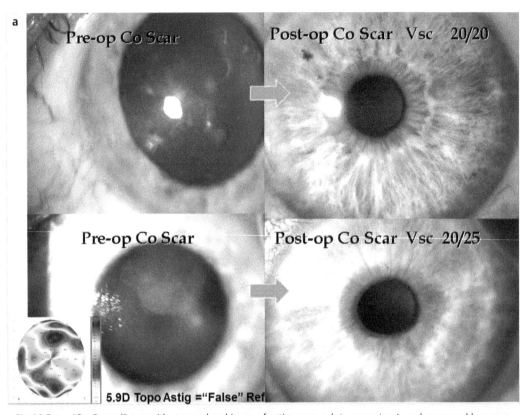

Fig. 16.5 a-c "On-Corneal" scar with scar peel and Laser refractive approach to emmetropia and measureable cornea. (*continued*)

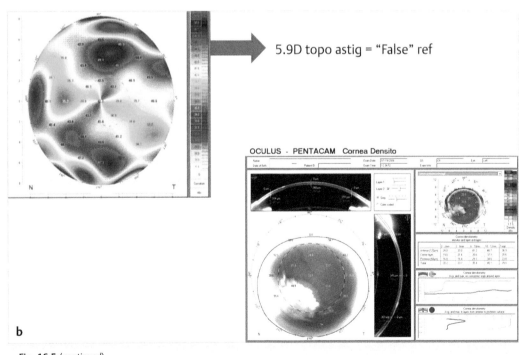

Fig. 16.5 (*continued*)

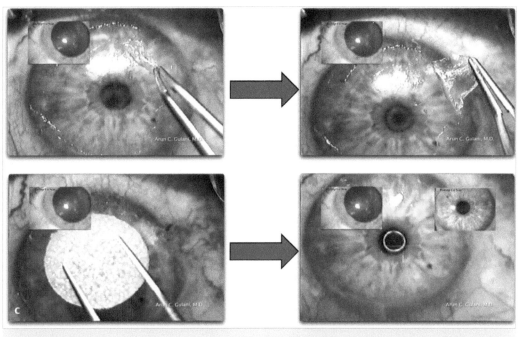

Fig. 16.5 (*continued*)

In some prototype cases, you shall see the application of these two categorical concepts to expand therewith the options and offerings to patients seeking a normal looking eye and in addition, seeing without glasses.[7]

In summary, we can apply unlimited applications, stages, or combinations to use full spectrum kerato-lenticulo-refractive techniques and technologies to either maintain vision or enhance it while aiming for a cosmetic outcome (▸ Fig. 16.6, ▸ Fig. 16.7, ▸ Fig. 16.8, ▸ Fig. 16.9, ▸ Fig. 16.10, ▸ Fig. 16.11, ▸ Fig. 16.12).

The importance of this procedure goes beyond successfully treating pterygium and pinguecula patients with a procedure that offers the opportunity for sparkling white eyes 1 day postoperatively to a long-term stability with a < 0.5% recurrence rate. It also offers a vehicle to maintain the integrity of the ocular surface—or further improve the ocular surface—thereby raising the bar on refractive surgery outcomes itself.

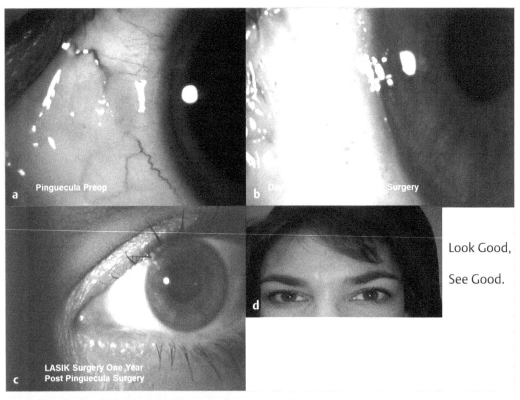

Fig. 16.6 (a-d) Look Good, See Good; Lasik surgery post pinguecula surgery.

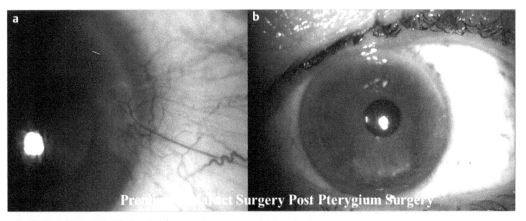

Fig. 16.7 (a,b) Look Good, See Good; cataract surgery post pterygium surgery.

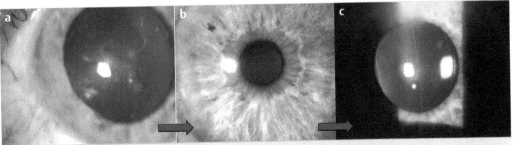

Fig. 16.8 (a-c) Advanced pterygium with scar clearance followed by toric IOL cataract surgery to 20/20. IOL, intraocular lens.

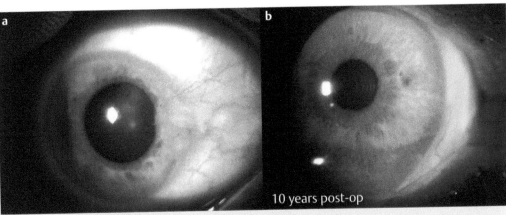

Fig. 16.9 (a,b) Pterygium surgery followed by multifocal IOL surgery to 20/20 and stable at 10 years. IOL, intraocular lens.

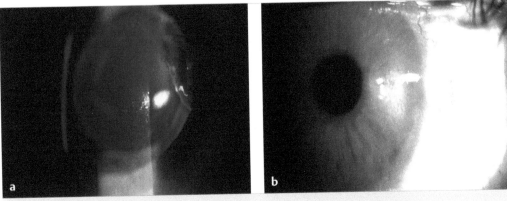

Fig. 16.10 (a,b) Maintaining 20/20 from previous Lasik and cataract surgery in a case of pterygium.

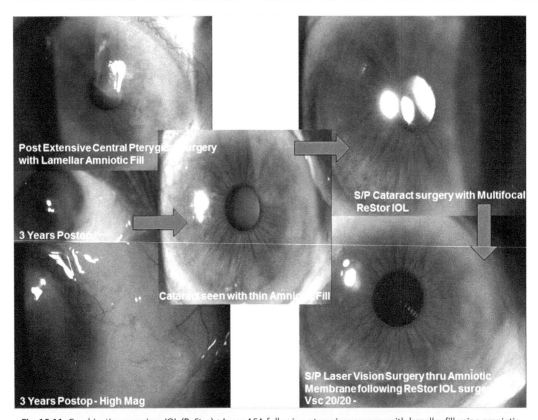

Fig. 16.11 Combination premium IOL (ReStor) + Laser ASA following pterygium surgery with lamellar fill using amniotic graft to 20/20 vision. ASA, advanced surface ablation; IOL, intraocular lens.

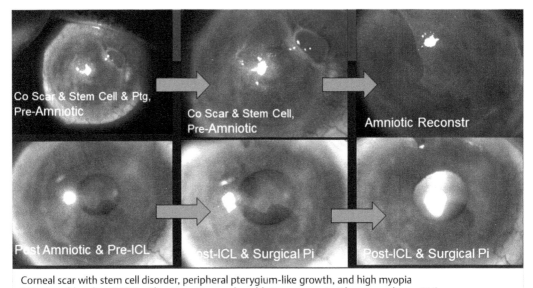

Corneal scar with stem cell disorder, peripheral pterygium-like growth, and high myopia (40-year-old male – 8.00D with astigmatism and unable to wear contact lenses or glasses OU) Post ICL: Vsc 20/25-OD (awaiting laser vision surgery) and Vsc 20/15 OS. Vsc = 20/15 OU distance and neare

Fig. 16.12 Pterygium like ocular surface surgery with AMT resulting in a measureable and stable cornea that allowed accurate ICL surgery to 20/25 unaided vision. Gulani-Tseng Collaboration. AMT, amniotic membrane transplantation; ASA, advanced surface ablation; ICL, implantable Collamer lens.

References

[1] Gulani A, Dastur YK. Simultaneous pterygium and cataract surgery. J Postgrad Med. 1995; 41(1):8–11

[2] Gulani AC. Corneoplastique: art of vision surgery. Indian J Ophthalmol. 2014; 62(1):3–11

[3] Gulani AC. Vision corrective surgeries: past techniques, present trends and future technologies. NEFM Journal of Medicine.. 2007; 2(58):41–44

[4] Gulani AC. Principles of surgical treatment of irregular astigmatism in unstable corneas. Text Book of Irregular Astigmatism. Diagnosis and Treatment. Thorofare, NJ: SLACK Incorporated; 2007:251–261

[5] Gulani AC. Evaluating the impact of femto laser-assisted capsulotomy. Cataract Refract Surg Today Europe. 2014; 9:36–50

[6] Gulani AC. Decoding corneal scars: Straight to 20/20. Ophthalmology Times.. 2014; 39(4):6–12

[7] Gulani AC. Shaping the future and reshaping the past: the art of vision surgery. Copeland and Afshari's Principles and Practice of Cornea. New Delhi, India: Jaypee Brothers Medical Publishers; 2013;2:1252–1273 [Chapter 98]

Index